The
Medicine Cabinet
of Curiosities

The
Medicine Cabinet
of Curiosities

An Unconventional Compendium
of Health Facts and Oddities,
from Asthmatic Mice
to Plants that Can Kill

Nicholas Bakalar

Times Books
Henry Holt and Company
New York

Times Books
Henry Holt and Company, LLC
Publishers since 1866
175 Fifth Avenue
New York, New York 10010
www.henryholt.com

Credits for the illustrations appear on pp. 211–12 as a continuation
of this page.

Library of Congress Cataloging-in-Publication Data

Bakalar, Nick.
  The medicine cabinet of curiosities : an unconventional
compendium of health facts and oddities, from asthmatic mice
to plants that can kill / Nicholas Bakalar.—1st ed.
      p. cm.
  Includes bibliographical references and index.
  ISBN-13: 978-0-8050-8854-0
  1. Medicine—Miscellanea.   I. Title.
  R706.B35   2009
  610—dc22   2009014739

Henry Holt books are available for special promotions and premiums.
For details contact: Director, Special Markets.

First Edition 2009
Designed by Meryl Sussman Levavi
Charts by Bob Roman

Printed in the United States of America

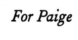

For Paige

CONTENTS

The
Medicine Cabinet
of Curiosities

INTRODUCTION

*The art of medicine consists of
amusing the patient while nature cures
the disease.*

—Voltaire (1694–1778)

DAILY CONVERSATION IS FILLED WITH HEALTH CHATTER, the more so as we age. Back pain, vitamins, infectious disease, amoxycillin, CAT scans, calcium, randomized studies, skipped heartbeats, MRIs, intravenous, low-fat, high-fiber, resistant germs, joint pain, vancomycin, ciprofloxacin, intramuscular, broad spectrum, narrow spectrum, urinary, digestive, flu, subcutaneous, tuberculosis, West Nile, Lyme disease—the vocabulary of health is infinite, the talk incessant, the opinions strong, the advice, both solicited and not, abundant. Part of this talk is even scientifically informed, although it is not always easy to know which part. *The Medicine Cabinet of Curiosities* is a random collection, put together with no more direction than that offered by the author's impulses, but it does

1

contain, so far as possible, just facts, and many of them, assembled in the hope that the reader's whims will at least occasionally coincide with those of the writer.

It should be needless to say, although it almost certainly is not, that there is in this book no medical advice whatsoever, and that anyone who uses it to diagnose or treat an illness, or to give advice based on its contents to others on how to do so, will be making a grave mistake.

There are citations to scientific papers and Web sites. We've made them into endnotes so that they are less distracting, but they are not there for decoration, or to give the text an air of authority that it might otherwise lack. They are there to prove that *The Medicine Cabinet* does not make anything up. And you still have to read them. Well, all right, you don't have to read them, but they're there if you want to, and you can always cite them in an argument.

This does not mean, we hasten to add, that there are no mistakes in this book. When you find one, as some of you no doubt will, please point it out. There is, however, no need to offer negative assessments of the author's intelligence, good faith, work habits, or ancestry, or to otherwise rub it in. All questioned facts will be carefully checked, and corrections will appear, duly noted and credited, in future editions.

This book is meant to be read in small doses, flipping from page to page at random, taking it up when the mood arrives and putting it down when it departs. It is arranged with this in mind, although we have divided it into sections, which we hope gives it a kind of organization, however vague the pattern and arbitrary the choice of headings. If you are looking for something specific, however, there is an index, which can be used in the usual way.

1

BY THE NUMBERS

*Doctors will have more lives to an-
swer for in the next world than even
we generals.*

—NAPOLEON I (1769–1821)

What Little Boys, Little Girls,
and All the Rest of Us Are Made Of

HYDROGEN, MOSTLY. IN ELEMENTARY SCHOOL YOU HEARD that we are 65 percent water, or something like that, right? As usual, you didn't get the full story. In reality, your body is 62.91 percent hydrogen, 24.003 percent oxygen, and 11.97 percent carbon—that's a little more than 98.89 percent of you, and we've only accounted for three elements. You're 0.58 percent nitrogen, 0.24 percent calcium, 0.14 percent phosphorus, and 0.04 percent sulfur, so those four make up about another 1 percent. That leaves roughly 11 one-hundredths of 1 percent for everything else. You are about 0.0000000000000015259 percent radium. That's 80 billion atoms—not very many.

Here's what a 155-pound man is made of, atom for atom:

Estimated Atomic Composition of the Lean 70-kg Male Human Body

Element	Sym	# of Atoms	Element	Sym	# of Atoms	Element	Sym	# of Atoms
Hydrogen	H	4.22×10^{27}	Rubidium	Rb	2.2×10^{21}	Zirconium	Zr	2×10^{19}
Oxygen	O	1.61×10^{27}	Strontium	Sr	2.2×10^{21}	Cobalt	Co	2×10^{19}
Carbon	C	8.03×10^{26}	Bromine	Br	2×10^{21}	Cesium	Cs	7×10^{18}
Nitrogen	N	3.9×10^{25}	Aluminum	Al	1×10^{21}	Mercury	Hg	6×10^{18}
Calcium	Ca	1.6×10^{25}	Copper	Cu	7×10^{20}	Arsenic	As	6×10^{18}
Phosphorus	P	9.6×10^{24}	Lead	Pb	3×10^{20}	Chromium	Cr	6×10^{18}
Sulfur	S	2.6×10^{24}	Cadmium	Cd	3×10^{20}	Molybdenum	Mo	3×10^{18}
Sodium	Na	2.5×10^{24}	Boron	B	2×10^{20}	Selenium	Se	3×10^{18}
Potassium	K	2.2×10^{24}	Manganese	Mn	1×10^{20}	Beryllium	Be	3×10^{18}
Chlorine	Cl	1.6×10^{24}	Nickel	Ni	1×10^{20}	Vanadium	V	8×10^{17}
Magnesium	Mg	4.7×10^{23}	Lithium	Li	1×10^{20}	Uranium	U	2×10^{17}
Silicon	Mg	3.9×10^{23}	Barium	Ba	8×10^{19}	Radium	Ra	8×10^{10}
Fluorine	F	8.3×10^{22}	Iodine	I	5×10^{19}			
Iron	Fe	4.5×10^{22}	Tin	Sn	4×10^{19}			
Zinc	Zn	2.1×10^{22}	Gold	Au	2×10^{19}			
Total		6.71×10^{27}						

The Smallest Bone in the Human Body

The stapes, one of three bones in the middle ear. It's also the lightest bone in the body and helps to transmit sound vibrations to the inner ear.

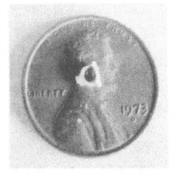

The stapes and a penny, larger than life.

The Biggest Bone in the Human Body

The femur, or thighbone, which runs from hip to knee. It's also the longest bone in the body and, if it's in good health, could support about thirty times your weight.

By a Hair's Breadth

"Smaller than the width of a human hair" is the description people sometimes use when they're trying to describe something really, really small. But what exactly is the width of a human hair?

It varies, for a number of reasons. Different people have different hair thicknesses. Dark hair tends to be thicker than light-colored hair. Babies have finer hair than adults. Age thickens some body hairs. And each hair varies in thickness from the root to the tip. So "the width of a human hair" is a pretty imprecise figure any way you look at it.

How imprecise? Very. A good estimate is that a human hair can vary in thickness from about 15 microns (a micron is 39 one-millionths of an inch) to about 180 microns. So, big deal, we say: what's a few millionths of an inch between friends? Well, not much, but one hair can be twelve times thicker than another. If you simply mean that something is very thin, then "the width of a human hair" is probably good enough. But what if someone asked you how tall something is and you replied "It's about as tall as a ladder"? Do you mean a five-foot stepladder or a sixty-foot fire truck extension beam? In most everyday situations, a few microns one way or the other doesn't make much difference, but if you're designing the display coating for a TV screen, the circuitry for an iPhone, or a lithium-ion battery for a laptop computer, you have to be a lot more precise than "the width of a human hair."

Losing Our Hair

Nonhuman primates, like most mammals, are covered with fur. So why is it that humans are the only (mostly) hairless ape? Darwin thought it was unlikely that hairlessness evolved by natural selection alone, since hair protects skin against the damaging rays of the tropical sun. Which makes it even more puzzling, as a matter of biology, when you consider where we do have hair—in our armpits, around our sexual organs, and on our heads.

A 1981 paper suggested that the answer has to do with heat dissipation. As the ratio of surface area to volume decreases, the advantage of having lots of insulation decreases, too. A 450-pound gorilla has a mass a thousand times that of a half-pound marmoset, but an exposed surface only a hundred times as great. So the great ape needs less fur to keep the heat in. When humans emerged from the forest to explore the open savannah, they developed hairlessness to allow heat to escape, and then sweat glands to cool their bodies by evaporation. The evolution of sweat glands allowed even more extensive hairlessness to evolve. Presumably the evolution of darker skin happened for the same reason. None of this, of course, explains the persistence of armpit and pubic hair.

A newer theory is that humans lost their hair to get rid of lice, fleas, and ticks and the diseases those animals carry, such as typhus, trench fever, and bubonic plague. This makes having less hair sexually attractive because it signals good health. And sexual attractiveness gives the trait survival value. Do we think this explains why women, and now increasingly men, want to rid their bodies of hair? Maybe. And then again, maybe not.

The Quick and the Dead

Fingernails and toenails are made of a protein called keratin, and the nails have several different parts, most of them with names you've probably never heard of. The eponychium, better known as the cuticle, is the piece of skin where the finger meets the bottom of the nail. The skin around the edges is called the paronychium. The hyponychium is the skin that connects underneath the tip of the nail. The nail plate is the part on top that you see and polish, and the nail bed—sometimes called the quick—is the tissue that's under the nail. The white half-moon at the bottom of your fingernail is called the lunula.

Fingernails grow about a tenth of an inch a month, toenails about three one-hundredths of an inch. They grow from the bottom out—the part that you file or clip is the oldest part, and it's dead. For some reason, nails grow faster in the summer than in the winter. They grow faster during pregnancy, but on the whole, men's grow faster than women's. And the nails on your dominant hand grow faster than those on the other hand.

Nails lose their water content with age, which can make them crack or peel. Living in a cold, dry climate and washing your hands a lot can also dry them out and cause cracking and peeling.

Nails can get fungal infections, which are more common

in the toenails than on the hands. Bacteria can infect the tissue around the nails, which often happens after an injury. Warts and tumors can appear around or under nails, and if a tumor is big enough, surgery may be required to remove it.

The longitudinal ridges you see in your nails are the result of aging, and don't suggest any health problem. However, although no doctor would depend on examining them to make a diagnosis, fingernails and toenails can sometimes suggest certain other health problems. Those white spots you occasionally see usually mean nothing—they're often caused by minor trauma to the ends of your fingers—but sometimes they can indicate an infection. Psoriasis can cause flattening of the nails, and certain thyroid and lung conditions can cause brittleness. Dark spots on the nails have to be looked at by a dermatologist—they can be a sign of melanoma, a deadly skin cancer. But if you have a serious health problem, your fingernails are not the first place you'll notice it, and they're not the first place a doctor will look, either.

The Smallest Surviving Baby

Records are imperfect, so it's hard to say exactly who holds claim to the title of smallest baby ever, but Amillia Sonja Taylor, born at Baptist Children's Hospital in Miami, Florida, on October 24, 2006, is the smallest for whom there is a reliable record. She was nine and a half inches long and weighed just under ten ounces after a gestation that lasted a little less than twenty-two weeks. She went home in February 2007 weighing four and a half pounds. In July 2007, according to a report in *People* magazine, she was healthy, weighed fourteen pounds three ounces, and was able to hold up her head and sit with support.

Vital Statistics

We are sorry to note that the percentage of preterm births—those at less than thirty-seven weeks' gestation—increased by 20 percent between 1990 and 2005.

Percentage of Births by Gestational Age

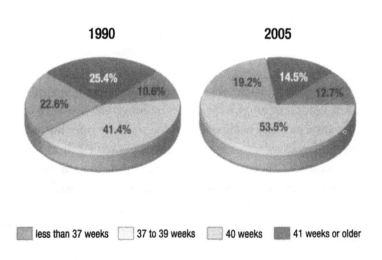

1990

25.4% 10.6% 22.6% 41.4%

2005

19.2% 14.5% 12.7% 53.5%

less than 37 weeks   37 to 39 weeks   40 weeks   41 weeks or older

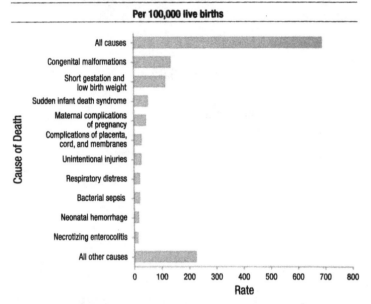

Mortality Rates for the Ten Leading Causes of Infant Death

The United States ranks just twenty-ninth in infant mortality, compared to twelfth in 1960, though the actual infant mortality rate has declined, to 6.9 deaths per one thousand live births. (Singapore ranks number one, with 2 deaths per one thousand births.) Congenital malformations, disorders related to low birth weight, and sudden infant death syndrome account for 43 percent of all infant deaths.

In Black and White

African Americans suffer more health problems than white Americans, and they often get poorer medical care. The problem is complicated, and racism and other prejudices are only sometimes a factor, but hundreds of studies have demonstrated a clear pattern in which white and black patients are treated differently. In any case, we consider the following highly disturbing:

In New York City, black babies with very low birth weights (less than three pounds five ounces) are more likely to be born in hospitals with high risk-adjusted neonatal death rates. Only 11 percent of white very low birth weight (VLBW) babies were born at hospitals with high death rates, while 21 percent of black VLBW babies were born at such hospitals.

Black patients get less opioid pain relief medicine than white people. According to Dr. Mark Pletcher of the University of California, San Francisco, this disparity was identified in the 1990s, and there was hope that a national campaign aimed "at improving pain management in emergency departments would shrink this disparity. . . . Unfortunately, this is not the case."

Black patients are less likely than white to receive various kinds of cancer therapy. A study finds that despite efforts in the last decade to mitigate cancer treatment disparities, black patients are significantly less likely than white patients to receive therapy for various types of cancer. Once again, efforts initiated in the 1990s to close treatment gaps appear to have had little impact.

African Americans wait longer than white people to receive kidney transplants. There are many reasons why some patients get organs faster than others, but an important one is match by race.

Black patients are less likely to receive mitral valve repairs, the treatment for mitral valve disease, a type of heart disease. African Americans present for mitral valve surgery at a significantly younger age than whites and with more risk factors, but they don't receive mitral valvuloplasty at the same

11

rates, even though the operation can have an effect on long-term outcome. The reasons are not clear.

Black patients are more likely to die from soft-tissue cancers than whites. This kind of cancer is rare, but it's very serious. Researchers studied 4,636 whites, 663 blacks, 696 Hispanics, and 411 Asians with the diagnosis. Blacks diagnosed with soft-tissue sarcomas in an arm or a leg were much less likely than other groups to receive certain limb-sparing treatments, and their overall survival was poorer. Blacks were 39 percent more likely to die from the disease, even when other factors are taken into account.

Black patients are less likely than whites to undergo thorough examination and surgery for treatable lung cancer, even when they have equal access to specialized medical care.

Blacks with chronic obstructive pulmonary disorder are less likely to undergo lung transplants than whites, even after controlling for age, lung function, pulmonary hypertension, obesity, and diabetes. Insurance, cardiovascular risk factors, and poverty explained part—but not all—of the differences in treatment.

Black smokers are less likely to be screened for tobacco use and less likely to be advised to quit. During visits to health care providers in 2007, 63 percent of white smokers were advised to quit smoking, while 55 percent of black smokers got the same recommendation. And it wasn't because the black smokers were poorer or had worse insurance factors—the researchers statistically accounted for those variables in their study.

When Medicare began paying for women to undergo preventive mammograms in 1991, doctors expected breast cancer mortality rates to drop. Breast cancer deaths did decrease, but not as quickly for African American women as a group—though breast cancer death rates for black and white women used to be nearly identical. And while breast cancer death rates are decreasing for white women in every U.S. state, for African American women, death rates are decreasing in only eleven of the thirty-seven states with sufficient numbers for analysis and in the District of Columbia. In the rest, death rates are either flat (twenty-four states) or increasing (in Arkansas and Mississippi).

Black patients are less likely to receive chemotherapy or radiation therapy for rectal cancer, though black patients and white patients see rectal cancer specialists at similar rates. African Americans were 23 percent less likely to receive chemotherapy for rectal cancer, and 12 percent less likely to receive radiation therapy, than whites. "We knew that African Americans were not receiving chemotherapy for rectal cancer at the same rates as white Americans and it was contributing to their increased mortality. Now we have a better idea of where the problem lies: somewhere between the visit with the oncologist and the actual initiation of chemotherapy," says Dr. Arden Morris of the University of Michigan Medical School and the Veterans Administration Ann Arbor Healthcare System.

Black patients are more likely to die in the early stages of chronic kidney disease.

Individual physicians achieve less favorable outcomes among their black diabetes patients than among their white patients. One factor is socioeconomic: poorer people have poorer outcomes, regardless of the seriousness of the disease. But there were still racial disparities in outcomes, and they were attributable not to differences between physicians or between health plans, but to individual physicians. According

Rate of Death, Adjusted by Age

Per 100,000 population

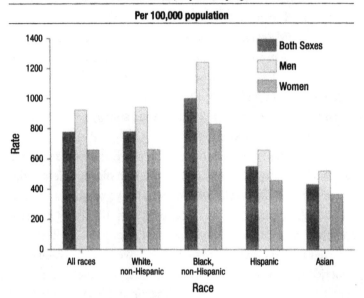

to this study, physicians treat black and white patients differently, and whites get better care.

Black males have the highest death rate—and a higher death rate across most of the leading causes of death.

2

BUTTERFLIES IN THE STOMACH

A skilful leech is better far, than half
a hundred men of war.

—Samuel Butler (1612–1680)

Real Diseases That Sound Like
They Were Invented for a Horror Movie

WE DON'T KNOW YOUR TASTE IN HORROR, BUT BLEEDING organs, bloody vomit, diarrhea that can kill you, flesh-eating bacteria, and the like seem a good bet.

Ebola hemorrhagic fever. First identified in 1976 in the Sudan and Zaire (what is now the Democratic Republic of the Congo) as two separate species of virus, Ebola is one of the most virulent viral diseases known. Of the 1,850 cases that have been documented by the World Health Organization, more than 1,200 of the people infected died. With mortality rates like that, it's no wonder it has already become the favored disease of thriller writers.

Ebola begins with a sudden fever, weakness, muscle pain, headache, and a bad sore throat. You then enter the vomiting, diarrhea, rash, red eyes, incessant hiccups, and kidney-and-liver-problem-so-you-can't-rest stage. Often there is bleeding, internally and externally. There's no vaccine, and there's no treatment other than trying to stay hydrated and comfortable.

Usually, outbreaks can be traced back to contact with infected animals—chimpanzees, gorillas, monkeys, forest antelopes—both dead and alive. It can also be transmitted from person to person, and direct contact with the corpse of someone who died from it will get you infected.

In 2007, an outbreak in Uganda infected 149 people, with 39 fatalities. To make this killer disease even more horrifying, scientists confirmed that a new species of the Ebola virus was the culprit. There are now four known species of Ebola.

Marburg hemorrhagic fever. It starts suddenly, with a high fever, bad headaches, muscle pain, and malaise. Within a day, you are rapidly becoming debilitated. On day three, you start vomiting, and you get severe watery diarrhea and terrible stomach pain. The diarrhea can last for a week, and you start to look really sick—drawn features, expressionless face, deep-set eyes. Some describe the patients as "ghostlike." Sometimes there's a rash, and few will find solace in the fact that it doesn't itch.

About day five, the bleeding starts. Blood in your feces, blood in your vomit, bloody nose, bloody gums, blood leaking out of your vagina (if you have one) or you get inflamed testicles (if you don't). High fever persists, and you become confused, irritable, and aggressive. After eight to nine days, you die, having suffered severe blood loss and shock. Sometimes, 75 percent of people affected live to tell the tale, but in a

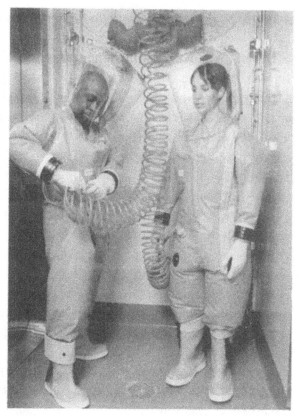

That's how nasty it is: suited up to work with Ebola.

2005 outbreak in Angola, mortality approached 100 percent. When the disease isn't fatal, recovery takes a long time, with continuing inflammations of the testes, the liver, the spinal cord, and the eyes. You can be infectious for up to seven weeks after you recover, and the virus can be transmitted in blood, urine, saliva, vomit, and respiratory mucus.

Marburg virus is a member of a family of viruses called filovirus, whose only other members are the species of Ebola. It is named after the German city where, in 1967, lab workers became ill with the virus after contact with African green monkeys that had been imported for research and to prepare polio vaccine. Around the same time, there were outbreaks in labs in Frankfurt and in Belgrade, but for some reason Marburg got the honor. (Infections have also been identified in South Africa, Kenya, and the Democratic Republic of the Congo.) When the disease isn't infecting humans, it apparently goes into hiding in monkeys.

Crimean-Congo hemorrhagic fever. Symptoms come on suddenly, with fever, aching muscles, dizziness, neck pain and stiffness, backache, headache, sore eyes, and painful sensitivity to light. Then there's the vomiting, diarrhea, sore throat, and general stomach pain. After that, the psychiatric symptoms start: sharp mood swings, confusion, irrational aggression. Apparently exhausted by this stage, you then become sleepy and depressed. That pain you feel in the upper right part of your abdomen is caused by liver enlargement.

And there are other symptoms as well, like a fast heartbeat and enlarged lymph nodes. Oh, yeah—the rash. Bleeding under the skin causes it, but you also get it inside your mouth and throat. Bloody feces, bloody nose, bloody urine, and bloody gums are additional features. Those who are really sick get liver, kidney, and lung failure after about five days, and one out of three is dead by the second week. The rest, after about ten days of agony, start to recover.

This tick-borne virus was first identified in the 1940s in the Crimea, but in 1956 the same virus turned up in the Congo, which explains its odd name.

Necrotizing fasciitis. Better known as "flesh-eating bacteria," this infection of the deep layers of skin kills about 50 percent of its victims. Several varieties of bacteria, including streptococci, have been involved—including since 2001 the now famous methicillin-resistant *Staphylococcus aureus* (MRSA).

The bacteria actually don't eat your flesh—or muscles or fat—but instead release a toxin that stimulates T-cells, the lymphocytes that play a role in fighting off diseases, which in turn activate cytokines. It's the cytokines that cause the tissue destruction.

Treatment involves aggressive surgical removal of affected tissue and intravenous antibiotics.

Fungal infiltration. Jock itch may be less terrifying than disgorging your blood and eating your flesh, but the idea of discovering full-blown mushrooms growing on your body is shiver-inducing. As recounted in *Mr. Bloomfield's Orchard*, by mycologist Nicholas Money, there have been cases of "ink-cap mushrooms growing in a patient's throat, a little bracket-forming basidiomycete in a gentleman's nose, dead babies covered in yeast, vaginal thrush gone wild, and a moldy penis." No wonder Money said the photographs of them "infected [his] nightmares for a month."

Worms That Live Inside You

There are several groups of multicellular organisms called helminths that can take up residence inside a human body, and all are revolting in their own way: flatworms, which include flukes and tapeworms; thorny-headed worms known as acanthocephala; roundworms, or nematodes, which can find refuge in human intestines or other tissue; and larva migrans, a real horror-movie favorite because it gets under the skin and crawls around there.

Flatworms are the simplest organisms that are bilaterally symmetrical—that is, they have matching right and left sides. Some are free-living, but the ones we're concerned with are the infamous parasitic tapeworms. Humans get these worms by eating their eggs.

Why would anyone eat the eggs of flatworms? Well, of course no one does so intentionally, but the worms are all over the world, and hatch eggs in food people do eat intentionally. There are various species that are transmitted to humans via fish (especially freshwater fish), pork, mutton, and beef.

The eggs can be seen either with the naked eye or under a microscope in the feces of infected people, and the unpleasant symptoms—abdominal distention, flatulence, cramping, and diarrhea—begin about ten days after you eat them. The way to diagnose the illness is to see the worms—usually the patient is instructed to collect feces samples in clean cardboard containers and to record the time each was collected. You have to collect several samples, because the flatworms shed in cycles and so they may appear in one sample but not in the next.

But the really bizarre part—and, let's face it, the part that a lot us find kind of amusing—is that after about a month, the larvae of some of these species mature into worms that can live for as long as ten years and reach lengths of up to thirty-two feet. The good news, at least under the circumstances, is that tapeworm infections can be treated with drugs and are rarely fatal. The drugs kill the adult organism, not the eggs, and if the worms migrate to other organs, like the liver or lungs, they may require surgical removal.

Thorny-headed worms have a proboscis that features curved hooks that conveniently attach to the tissue of their hosts. When humans are infected, it's very unpleasant. In 2008, researchers reported a case of a two-year-old girl in Iran who had been infected, probably by accidentally ingesting infected insects. She'd had mild stomach problems for about three months. The worms she had, which appeared repeatedly in her feces, were about five inches long and a tenth of an inch wide, and the proboscis was equipped with fourteen rows of six to eight curved hooks. Her worms were eliminated by treatment with a drug called mebendazole, which is sold under various brand names, including Ovex, Vermox, and Antiox. There are a half dozen species of these roundworms, also called intestinal roundworms, and at least one of them, *Enterobius vericularis*, or the pinworm, is fairly common in children in the United States. It is transmitted in feces—by kids who touch feces and each other, or adults who don't wash their hands properly after changing a child's diapers. Most infections are asymptomatic, but they can cause itching around the anus and vagina, plus vague symptoms of restlessness or intermittent nausea and other gastrointestinal problems.

Another kind of roundworm, called tissue roundworms, can also infect humans. Among these is the old favorite *Trichinella spiralis*, the cause of trichinosis, found in pork and beef. It causes the usual collection of unpleasant symptoms—nausea, diarrhea, vomiting, abdominal pain, and fever, plus a few extras like headaches, chills, eye swelling, aching joints, itchy skin, and muscle pain. There are a few other species common in other areas of the world, including *Onchorcerca volvulus*, the worm that causes river blindness, a disease that blinds about 300,000 people a year, almost all in Africa.

Finally, the larva migrans. There are two kinds, the creeping eruption caused by *Ancylostoma braziliense* and visceral larva migrans due to *Toxocara canis* and *Toxocara cati*. Creeping eruption causes itching, blisters, and raised snakelike tracks along the skin as the organism moves around. It can be treated with drugs, or it can go away by itself over a period of weeks or months. It's not common, except in tropical countries. Visceral larva migrans, on the other hand, has worldwide distribution, and besides taking residence in humans it also, as the Latin names suggest, lives in other mammals, including dogs and cats. While mild infections cause no symptoms, more serious infections can cause abdominal pain, cough, fever, and wheezing. Fortunately, it usually goes away by itself.

Maggot Therapy

The U.S. Food and Drug Administration (FDA) doesn't like maggots very much when they turn up in, say, canned tomatoes—although it has to find two or more per five hundred grams (a little more than seventeen ounces) before it deems the product repulsive enough to forbid its sale. Nevertheless, the agency finds them excellent for treating wounds, and it approved them as a medical device in January 2004. Doctors apply blowfly larvae—*Phaenicia sericata*, commonly called green bottle flies—to help heal pressure ulcers, venous stasis ulcers, neuropathic foot ulcers, and wounds from trauma or surgery that don't heal by themselves. In its Product Classification Database, the FDA calls them "Maggots, Medical," which has a nice ring to it.

There are records of using maggots on wounds that date back to the sixteenth century, and in his memoirs, Baron Dominique-Jean Larrey, one of Napoleon's surgeons, vividly describes how the men arriving at his field hospital with maggot-infested wounds healed more quickly. There is also a

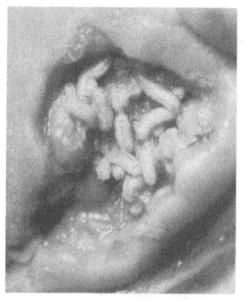

We know you just had to see some maggots in a wound.

large body of modern scientific literature testifying to their benefits. Maggots are used on wounds that have failed to heal by other means. They work very well at eating up dead tissue, cleansing, and disinfecting.

The larvae of green bottle flies need a moist environment with an ample source of nutrition—decaying animal carcasses are good, as are moist wounds. When the eggs hatch, the larvae immediately begin to secrete enzymes that liquefy decaying tissue and make it digestible. After they have eaten for four or five days, the maggots leave the wound (or rotting corpse) to find a dry place to enter their next phase of life, as pupae. The pupae hatch into adult flies. For medical purposes, technicians have the flies lay eggs in pork livers; then they remove the eggs and sterilize them. Sterile maggots are born from these sterile eggs.

A vial of 250 to 500 disinfected larvae costs $98 from a

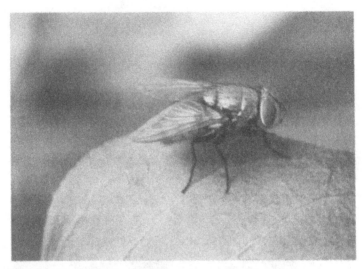

The maggot, medical, all grown up.

California company called Monarch Labs. There's a $41 charge for FedEx, which is the only way the company will ship them. It also sells sterile dressings, called "Creature Comforts," to be used with them. A prescription is required, and you're not allowed to use the larvae to breed your own, in case that's what you were planning.

Leech Me

Leeches are known to have been used by the Egyptians more than five thousand years ago for the treatment of various illnesses and conditions. They have been used ever since, with varying results, and in June 2004 the FDA finally approved their use for medicinal purposes, saying that they "can help heal skin grafts by removing blood pooled under the graft and restore blood circulation in blocked veins by removing pooled blood."

The animals secrete various substances in their saliva, including anti-inflammatories, vasodilators, anesthetics (a leech bite is usually painless), and several chemicals that inhibit blood clotting, the chief one of which is called hirudin, after the scientific name of the medicinal leech, *Hirudo medicinalis*. There are more than six hundred species of leech, ranging in size from a few centimeters to eighteen inches. Medical leeches run in the two- to four-inch range.

Leeches are used mainly in reconstructive microsurgery, aiding in the salvage of tissue in reattached fingers, ears, lips, and the tips of noses. There is good evidence that survival of the tissue is improved by the early application of a leech. The leech's saliva helps to move blood to tissue that has been deprived of it—like that detached finger. There can be complications, including infection, blood loss, allergic reactions, and the possibility that a leech can get lost in a body orifice or cavity. Unsurprisingly, there can also be significant adverse psychological consequences.

Leeches applied to wounds feed for about thirty minutes, and then they're full. They usually don't have to eat again for many months, but in any case, medicinal leeches are only used once—after that, they're medical waste, incinerated along with used needles, sponges, bandages, and the discarded tissue that winds up in those red containers in hospitals and doctors' offices.

There are anticlotting drugs like heparin that can be used, but leeches have some advantages over the artificial stuff. They aren't affected by the body's tendency to neutralize heparin with a substance called platelet factor 4, which is released as the body tries to stop the bleeding by coagulation, and they don't affect other enzyme pathways the way heparin does.

There are several companies that sell leeches for medical use. The one that submitted its product to the FDA and got approval is called Ricarimpex, and it's been around for 150 years. There's one in Wales, Biopharm Leeches, that takes as its corporate motto "The Biting Edge of Science." In the United States, Niagara Medical Leeches, Inc., sells leeches for $8 each, or $7 if you buy a hundred or more. It's $25 for shipping, no matter how many you buy, and you can order them online.

Bloodletting

Bloodletting has been used since antiquity and was widely practiced through the late nineteenth century—without much evidence that it worked. The idea was that removing large quantities of blood would somehow balance the humors—blood, phlegm, black bile, and yellow bile—and thus restore health. Needless to say, no one believes this anymore.

But bloodletting (the medical, and less colorful, term is "phlebotomy") is used to treat a few diseases, including hemochromatosis, a hereditary condition characterized by defective iron metabolism that causes an overload of iron in the body's tissues. This can lead to various kinds of organ damage, especially to the liver and pancreas. The treatment is to take blood out, and people with the disease usually schedule a blood donation one to four times a year. They also have to maintain a diet low in red meat and vitamin C and high in tea and calcium. The disease is fairly common—about 1 in 272 people in the United States have it, and that adds up to about a million people with the illness.

People with polycythemia, an abnormality of the bone marrow that results in an overproduction of red blood cells, are also treated with phlebotomy to keep their red blood count within normal limits. Polycythemia is a chronic disease of unknown origin that can have life-threatening complications such as stroke; it can also evolve into more serious illnesses including leukemia. It is a fairly rare disease, with an incidence of about 2.3 per 100,000. The median age at diagnosis is sixty.

Evil Doctors and Nurses

The simultaneous presence of sick people, old people, and poisonous drugs is apparently an irresistible temptation for mass murderers. Here are just a few egregious and terrifying examples.

Where there's a will. In 2000, Dr. Harold Shipman was found guilty of murdering fifteen people, but the prosecutors in the case said that there was probably enough evidence to prove that he killed as many as 250.

Most of Shipman's victims were women, and most were in good health. At one point, Shipman was almost caught, when the director of a funeral home, suspicious of the large number of cremations the doctor was signing off on, called in the police. But the investigators didn't find enough evidence to bring charges. Then, apparently, Shipman got greedy: he killed a woman named Kathleen Grundy, whose will left nothing to

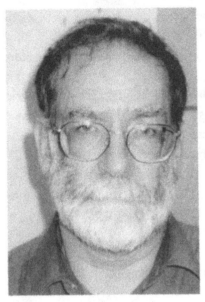

You probably weren't one of Dr. Harold Shipman's patients. If you were, congratulations.

her daughter and her daughter's children but gave £386,000 to Shipman. The police decided there was enough cause to dig up the body, and when they did, they found traces of heroin, a drug used (legally in Britain) for controlling pain in terminal cancer patients. Then they discovered that the will had been drawn up on a typewriter that was the same brand as the one Shipman owned. Shipman was arrested, and the police began to look into other patient deaths. It took a jury six days to convict him of the fifteen murders with which he was charged. Shipman never explained his motive. In fact, he never even confessed to the crimes, and he never will, because he committed suicide in prison in 2004.

A battery of evidence. Michael Swango was a guy someone should have caught on to early on, but no one did. Swango was an intern or resident at several different hospitals who is suspected of having killed at least sixty people over a fourteen-year period in the 1980s and 1990s. In 1984, when he was an intern at Ohio State University Hospital, three people claim they saw him inject something into a patient's IV just before she had a life-threatening seizure. There were four unexplained deaths during Swango's rotation on the neurosurgery ward there, but Swango claimed he'd done nothing wrong.

But trouble seemed to follow him. While working for an ambulance company in Illinois as a paramedic, he poisoned some iced tea with arsenic, which several of his colleagues drank. He was convicted of battery in the incident and spent the next two years in jail.

After his release, he somehow managed to get into a residency program in internal medicine at the University of South Dakota. He apparently managed to convince them that he was the victim of false accusations made by jealous coworkers. Then Swango applied for admission to the American Medical Association, and, noticing the felony conviction, the AMA mentioned it to the dean of the University of South Dakota medical school. They had the good sense to dismiss him from the residency program.

You would think that would be pretty much the end of it, but you'd be wrong. He next convinced the faculty of the medical school of the State University of New York at Stony Brook that the felony conviction was the result of a barroom brawl. So they admitted him to a residency in psychiatry. But then the dean at South Dakota found out Swango was still around and called the dean at SUNY to tell him that maybe Swango shouldn't be working there. The SUNY dean agreed and fired him.

Then Swango started forging his records to get jobs in other hospitals. When the hospitals found out who he was, they usually fired him, but he always managed to find a job somewhere else. Finally, spurred by an FBI investigation, he began seeking work in foreign countries. On his way to Saudi Arabia in June 1997, he was arrested for fraud, tried, convicted, and sentenced to forty-two months in prison.

In 1999, Ohio State University conceded that they should have called in investigators back in 1984, but by this time Swango's killing spree had spread to hospitals in Virginia, New York, and Zimbabwe. Finally, he agreed to plead guilty to three poisonings in New York in exchange for avoiding the death penalty. Zimbabwe wants to extradite him, but he's still in jail in New York.

Nursed to death. Nurse Charles Cullen killed his first patient—a judge who suffered from an allergic reaction to blood-thinning medicine—at St. Barnabas Medical Center in Livingston, New Jersey, in 1988.

Cullen left St. Barnabas in 1992, but not before killing eleven more patients with overdoses of various medicines. Cullen then got a job at Warren Hospital in Phillipsburg, New Jersey, where he killed three older women with overdoses of digoxin, a heart medicine. After a series of jobs in New Jersey—in 1997 he was fired from one hospital for incompetence—he got a license to practice nursing in Pennsylvania. He eventually settled at Easton Hospital in Easton, Pennsylvania, where he murdered another patient with digoxin. The hospital conducted an investigation, but no one suggested Cullen had anything to do with it.

Nurses are almost always in demand, though, and he landed a new job at Lehigh Valley Hospital in Allentown. There he killed one patient and allegedly attempted to kill another. He left that hospital under his own steam, took another job at St. Luke's Hospital in Bethlehem, and continued his spree with five more murders over the next three years. Coworkers complained that he always seemed to be around when people were dying, but still another investigation was inconclusive.

His next stop was Somerset Medical Center in Somerset, New Jersey. He was found asking for various medicines that hadn't been prescribed and going into the rooms of patients he wasn't assigned to. The New Jersey Poison Information and Education System warned Somerset Medical Center that at least four suspicious overdoses made them think an employee might be killing people. Somerset fired Cullen—not for killing people but for lying on his employment application.

Finally, in 2003, Cullen was arrested for and confessed to one murder and one attempted murder at Somerset Medical Center. He eventually pleaded guilty to killing twenty-two patients and attempting to kill five more. Cullen said he killed people in order to save them from further suffering. He is serving eleven consecutive life sentences in a prison in New Jersey.

Technically illegal. In 2007, a thirty-one-year-old man named Karl Helge Hampus Svensson was admitted to the Karolinska Institute, the prestigious Swedish medical school. A few months later, two anonymous letters arrived at the institute claiming that Svensson was a Nazi sympathizer who had been paroled from a maximum-security prison after serving time for murder. The letters turned out to be accurate.

After a trade union worker named Björn Söderberg complained that a colleague was expressing neo-Nazi beliefs at the workplace, the man, a friend of Svensson, had been fired. In 1999, Svensson had gotten into a loud argument with Söderberg outside his apartment in a Stockholm suburb, eventually shooting Söderberg seven times and killing him. Svensson served more than six years of an eleven-year sentence before being paroled. During his time in prison, he took academic courses, and on his release he interviewed for admission to the medical school. No one asked him about what he'd been doing for the previous seven years.

The institute couldn't think of a legal reason to expel him—there was no law in Sweden that said a murderer couldn't become a doctor, and he was not clearly a threat to others or suffering from a psychiatric illness. While some doctors, students, and officials argued that the man had served his time and was presumably rehabilitated, others said that a murderer, even a reformed one, should not be allowed to become a doctor.

Finally, the school nailed him on a technicality—they found out that he had changed the name on his high school transcript from Hellekant, the name he was convicted under, to Svensson, which he began using after being convicted of the crime. He was expelled in January 2008.

Unpleasant Things That Happen to the Human Body at High Altitude

No one can predict how you will be affected by high altitude. Being physically fit means nothing. It makes no difference whether you've been in training for the marathon for the past six months or spent that time sitting on your couch watching TV and eating potato chips. The only reliable predictor of how you will do in thin air is how you've done in the past. Therefore, if you've never been at high altitude before, flying in to Cuzco, Peru (altitude 11,000 feet), La Paz, Bolivia (altitude 11,300 feet), or Lhasa, Tibet (altitude 12,500 feet), can be a novel and very upsetting experience.

As altitude increases, atmospheric pressure decreases. As oxygen pressure decreases, you become hypoxic—unable to get enough oxygen for normal breathing. Not getting enough oxygen with each breath makes you breathe faster. This gets more oxygen into you, but it also causes respiratory alkalosis—a rise in blood pH level—that leads to dizziness, like you get from hyperventilating even at low altitudes (but you don't need to try it out now). No one is quite sure of the exact mechanisms, but apparently the cells in your body start to accumulate sodium and water and expel potassium. This makes the cells swell—what is commonly called water retention. Then your body tries to compensate for this abnormal condition by expelling urine. This helps, but not enough. You're getting the first and most mild form of altitude illness, called acute mountain sickness (AMS).

This doesn't happen right away; it usually takes several hours at high altitude—as low as 4,000 feet, but usually after quick ascent to around 9,000 feet—before your symptoms appear. You get a headache and start to feel very tired. You lose your appetite and feel nauseous. You might vomit. If your reactions don't get too severe, you start to get accustomed to the altitude, and the symptoms begin to disappear after a few days.

If you don't get better, the next stage is high-altitude pulmonary edema (HAPE). Now fluid is starting to leak into your lungs—it's as if you're starting to drown. You're gasping for breath every time you try to move, and eventually even when you're standing still. Sometimes you cough up bloody sputum. You have noisy breathing that sounds like you've got pneumonia. Your skin takes on a pale bluish tinge, and you get a fever. If the breathlessness goes on at rest for more than a few minutes, you're in real trouble, and you have to descend to a lower altitude. If you don't, you move to the most dangerous stage of altitude sickness: high-altitude cerebral edema (HACE).

You officially have HACE if you fail the "tandem gait test." This is the heel-to-toe walking exercise the police sometimes use to see if a driver is drunk. Your brain is starting to swell because of the accumulation of fluid in and around your brain cells. This makes you lose control of your muscles. You get confused and start to have hallucinations, and you have a colossal headache. Unless you're moved to lower altitude within a few hours after the first symptoms appear, you go into a coma. Then you die.

All this can be prevented by ascending slowly, by spending about two days moving from sea level to 8,000 feet and then a day for every 2,000 feet higher. Drinking lots of water is a good idea, too, because dehydration makes symptoms worse. Alcohol is bad; frequent small carbohydrate-rich meals are good. "Water pills"—such as acetazolamide (brand name Diamox)—are a good preventive for AMS.

And keep in mind that there are no permanent residents above 18,000 feet, except dead ones.

Equally Unpleasant Things That Happen to the Human Body in Very Deep Water

And sometimes not even all that deep.

Snorkelers sometimes purposely hyperventilate: you force several fast, deep breaths before you hold your breath for a dive in order to increase the amount of time you can stay underwater. This works because hyperventilation increases the amount of air entering the alveoli in your lungs and reduces the carbon dioxide pressure in your blood. Thus, it takes longer for the carbon dioxide to build up to the point where you have to take a fresh breath of air.

However, the technique doesn't increase the amount of oxygen in the blood, which falls. In a dive, even a relatively shallow one, the pressure of the water increases the pressure of gases in the lungs, including oxygen, allowing sufficient oxygen pressure to be maintained even though there's less oxygen available. When, eager for a breath, you start to surface, the lowering pressure of the surrounding water makes the oxygen pressure in your lungs decrease as well. Now you not only don't have enough oxygen, but you don't have enough oxygen pressure, either. That combination can make you pass out as you surface.

Scuba divers don't have this problem, because the equipment delivers oxygen under the same pressure as the surrounding water. With enough oxygen at the right pressure you can stay underwater for extended periods of time—but not too extended. The increased effort that breathing takes under high pressure can wear a diver out quickly.

Other bad things can happen, too. If the scuba gear's oxygen pressure is too great—about one and a half times the pressure at the surface—it can give rise to convulsions or make fluid leak into your lungs.

And then there is the threat of nitrogen narcosis, or "rapture of the deep." While you are scuba diving, you are breathing air at a pressure equal to the pressure of the water around you. Air is about 78 percent nitrogen, so you're breathing nitrogen at increased pressure, too. Nitrogen is absorbed by fatty tissue faster than by other tissue, and the brain and nervous system are full of fatty tissue. If too much nitrogen gets absorbed, the brain doesn't function properly, and you become mentally impaired. Sometimes you experience a feeling of light-headed euphoria; sometimes you start to act irrationally. If it gets really bad, you go into convulsions and pass out. This can start to happen at depths as shallow as thirty feet. If you keep your wits about you and are able to surface properly, the problem goes away.

But surfacing properly is a problem, too. If you surface too quickly, the gases that have been dissolved in your tissue begin to bubble out, expanding as the water pressure decreases. Unless they are gradually vented, you suffer decompression sickness, sometimes called caisson disease or the bends. You start to take very rapid shallow breaths and get arm or leg joint pain, which can become very severe. There's usually no joint inflammation, and the pain isn't affected by movement. About half the time, you get neurological problems as well, ranging from tingling sensations in the extremities to major brain problems. If the spinal cord gets involved, you can suffer irreversible paralysis. The treatment is 100 percent oxygen, and recompression followed by gradual decompression.

Can Your Hair Turn Gray Overnight?

The short answer: no. Hair gets its color from melanin, the same substance that darkens skin. There are two pigment types involved: eumelanin, for dark colors including brown, and pheomelanin, for reddish and yellow colors. The pigment moves from the cells that produce it, called melanocytes, to the keratinocytes that make up hair. Keratinocytes die and retain their color—your hair is dead as a doornail despite what all those TV ads say about lively, glowing, vivid, shining locks.

When the melanocytes stop producing pigment, your hair

loses color. Gray hair has less pigment, white hair none at all. Hair color is controlled by genes, so some people go gray earlier, some later, and some not at all. The rule of thumb is that among Caucasians, half are half-gray by age fifty. For other ethnic groups, the proportions vary. But however it happens, and for whatever reasons, graying is a gradual process, and doesn't happen overnight.

3

X, Y, AND SEX

*The great secret of doctors, known
only to their wives, but still hidden
from the public, is that most things
get better by themselves; most things,
in fact, are better in the morning.*

—LEWIS THOMAS (1919–1993)

How Not to Improve Your Sex Life

IN JANUARY 2008, THE FOOD AND DRUG ADMINISTRATION issued a list of "dietary supplements" being sold in stores or on the Internet as cures for erectile dysfunction. Many of these products are sold with labels suggesting that they are "all-natural" and therefore safe alternatives to prescription drugs; some are totally ineffective. In some cases, the supplements even contained prescription drugs or other potentially harmful ingredients without appropriate notice and warnings. Among the ingredients the FDA found were sildenafil and vardenafil, the active ingredients in, respectively, Viagra and Levitra, two FDA-approved prescription drugs for the treatment of erectile dysfunction. If a person is taking drugs containing nitrates for other medical conditions, these ingredients can lower blood pressure to unsafe levels.

Actra-Rx

Actra-Sx

Libidus

Nasutra

Neophase

Vigor-25

Yilishen

Zimaxx

4EVERON

Liviro3

Lycium Barbarum L.

Adam Free

Rhino V Max

V.Max

True Man

Energy Max

HS Joy of Love

NaturalUp

Blue Steel

Erextra

Super Shangai

Strong Testis

Shangai Ultra

Shangai Ultra X

Lady Shangai

Shangai Regular, also
marketed as Shangai
Chaojimengnan

Hero

The FDA says that the number of these products is increasing, so you can be pretty sure this list is incomplete.

Sometimes the FDA is able to get a manufacturer to voluntarily stop selling a pill or to recall it. In fact, in May 2008, the agency requested that a company recall a pill that didn't make its earlier list—Xiadafil VIP Tabs—because it contained a "potentially harmful, undeclared ingredient that may dangerously affect a person's blood pressure and can cause other life-threatening side effects." The hazardous ingredient is an analogue of sildenafil.

The FDA's advice is not to buy these supplements. Our advice is that if you do buy them, don't swallow them.

50 Percent

We don't think fifty-fifty is good odds. According to the Centers for Disease Control and Prevention (CDC), at least 50 percent of sexually active men and women get the human papillomavirus (HPV) at some point in their lives, and women in their twenties have the highest rate of infection. Infection with HPV increases women's risk for cervical cancer.

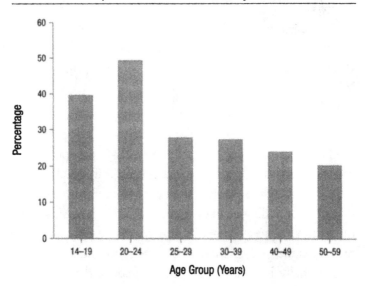

Human Papillomavirus Infection in Sexually Active Women

Why Do Men—and Sometimes Women, Too—
Go Bald?

Androgenetic alopecia—male pattern baldness—afflicts about two-thirds of men by the time they're sixty years old. In this kind of baldness, the hairs along the midline of the scalp get smaller and smaller, to the point where they disappear completely, and the scalp line recedes, all the way to the back of the neck in some men. The balding is caused by an increased sensitivity of the hairs to the effects of the male hormone, testosterone.

For a while, people blamed mothers for passing along the genes for male pattern baldness. Then for a while, the father started getting the blame. Now a group of German geneticists believe they have found the gene that is largely responsible for the phenomenon, at least when it happens early in life. It's an androgen receptor gene, and androgen-related genes are critical in developing masculine characteristics. But here's the catch: it's located on the X chromosome, so we're cursing the maternal line after all.

But it's also for this reason that women, too, sometimes experience androgenetic alopecia—though not as often and usually not as severely. The cause: increased levels of circulating androgens, which come from the ovaries or the adrenal glands, most often after menopause.

If you have no evidence of a severe imbalance in androgen hormones, then there are two effective drug treatments for your baldness: the topical application of liquid minoxidil (Rogaine) or a pill called finasteride (Propecia, Proscar). Rogaine is approved for both men and women, but finasteride is approved only for men because it causes birth defects and its safety and effectiveness in women haven't been established in

41

clinical trials. (Women, the manufacturers warn, aren't even supposed to touch the stuff.) These drugs are effective because the follicles that produce hair don't die in androgenetic alopecia—given the right stimulus they can start producing hair again.

Propecia and Proscar are actually the same drug, but Propecia—for growing more hair—comes in one-milligram tablets, and Proscar—for reducing the size of an enlarged prostate—comes in five-milligram tablets. You have to take your Propecia pill every day; if you stop taking it, your hair stops growing, and you wind up just as bald as you ever were. Same is true for minoxidil—you have to keep rubbing it in for the rest of your life if you want to keep your hair on your head. Minoxidil is off patent, so you can buy a cheaper generic form. Finasteride is also off patent as a treatment for benign prostatic hyperplasia, but Merck holds a patent on its use as a hair-growing medicine in the United States until 2013.

There are other causes of baldness. There's a type called telogen effluvium in which normal hairs start to shed as a result of environmental or systemic stresses. A change in hormones, especially the kind that sometimes occurs after a woman gives birth, can also cause hair to start dropping out. In healthy people, hairs grow, die, and fall out at different times, so that there are always younger hairs growing to replace the older ones. But under these kinds of stresses, the hairs start growing synchronously, and therefore they die and fall out at the same time. This kind of hair loss stops by itself when the stress disappears, and the hair grows back without treatment.

In alopecia areata, the hair falls out in circular patches, separated by areas of hair growth. In severe cases, the separate areas connect, resulting in total baldness. This can happen when the growth areas around the hair follicles get surrounded by T lymphocytes, a type of white blood cell. This is usually caused by disease such as hyperthyroidism, hypothyroidism, or vitiligo, a chronic skin disease. It can also happen to people with Down syndrome.

Sometimes a parasite can cause baldness. Usually, the parasite is *Trichophyton tonsurans*, a fungus that grows on skin. There are oral medicines and shampoos that can get rid of the stuff, but you have to examine family members and close associates of anyone who has an infestation—it can travel from one person to another by close contact.

Hair loss can also be caused by mechanical means—pulling it out with the misuse of curlers, rubber bands, or overly tight braiding. The solution to this problem is to change your hairstyle. There's a psychological disorder called trichotillomania, in which a person compulsively pulls out his or her hairs. For this, psychotherapy or treatment with antidepressants, or both together, can be effective.

Why Do Women Live Longer than Men?

It's true of most animal species: the females live longer than the males. This probably has something to do with sexual selection. Males have to compete for females, so they tend to put large amounts of energy into that competition—peacocks grow huge tails and deer grow big antlers, which expends energy; and the males of many species fight over females, which can result in injury and early death. Because successful breeders don't tend to live long, there's no selection for longevity among the males of these species. Natural selection doesn't maximize life span; it maximizes the chance that genes will be passed on to the next generation. If the successful transmission of genes requires that an animal die young, natural selection doesn't really care.

But if that explains anything, it doesn't explain the problem in humans, where men don't habitually get into physical fights over women and don't grow large decorations to impress them. Yet it has been true since as long as anyone can determine—and researchers have gone back as far as the fourteenth century—that women live longer than men. Throughout the twentieth century, the gap widened, as infectious disease became less a cause of death and other causes became more prominent: weapons, accidents with automobiles and other machinery, tobacco, alcohol, and other drugs, all of which affect men more than women. In other words, whatever evolutionary reasons there are for men's shorter life span, they interact with cultural adaptations.

Men die more than women at every age. More boys than girls are born, but the boys start dying quite young, even in childhood. Young men pursue risky strategies (see "Why Teenagers Act Nuts" in chapter 11), and they die in accidents much more often than young women do. As people age, in every age group, more men than women die from cancer, heart disease, and other ailments.

The discrepancy between men and women is greater among lower socioeconomic groups and the unmarried. Some researchers suggest that men with fewer resources have to take greater risks, leading to higher mortality rates. And some men believe that adopting risky strategies enhances their reproductive success.

Life Expectancy at Birth

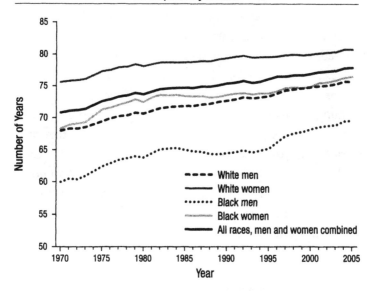

Why Women Get More Cavities than Men

Okay, so women live longer, but they have to spend some of that extra time in the dentist's chair, so maybe it's not such a bargain.

Apparently women have had more dental problems for quite a long time. A University of Oregon anthropologist, John Lukacs, reviewed studies of the frequency of cavities in both living and prehistoric populations around the world and consistently found that women have more rotten teeth than men.

He concluded that there are a number of biological reasons for this, including women's preadolescent sex hormones, menstrual cycles, and hormonal fluctuations. When women are pregnant, they experience more hormone fluctuations, their saliva composition changes, they have diet changes and possibly diet cravings, and their immune systems are suppressed. All of this helps to increase tooth decay. In studies of old skeletons, researchers found evidence of a strong correlation between agriculture and tooth decay. When people started farming, women started becoming pregnant more often— and because pregnancy affects women's oral health, they also started losing their teeth more often.

Even though girls tend to have more cavities than boys, Lukacs concludes, it's really pregnancy that makes teeth rot. The old wives' tale that you lose a tooth for every child may not be far from the truth.

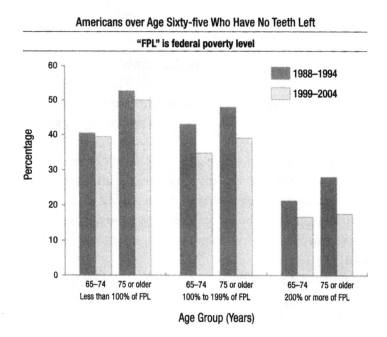

Americans over Age Sixty-five Who Have No Teeth Left

Rotten Luck

The poor aren't lucky in many ways, including that on average they have fewer teeth.

Will It Be a Boy or a Girl?

Are some people more likely to be parents of girls than boys? Yes. Why? It's in their genes—at least, that is, in the men's genes.

Some patient and diligent researchers read through 927 family trees that included information on 556,387 North Americans and Europeans to see who had boys and who had girls. The data went as far back as the early seventeenth century. They found that some men—but not women—have a gene that makes them produce more boys, a gene that is transmitted to their sons but not their daughters. So the sons, but not the daughters, of the men who have this boy-producing gene are also more likely to produce boys than girls.

This finding helps explain a rather strange phenomenon. After large wars, when lots of men are killed, the number of boys born rises. Some have attributed this to divine intervention, but apparently there is a more earthly explanation.

Here's what apparently happens. Suppose you have two families. Each has five children. The first family has two sons, but the other—because the father has the boy-producing gene—has five. Off the boys go to war, and in each family one son gets killed. That eliminates 50 percent of the sons from the family whose father lacks the gene, but only 20 percent of the sons from the family whose father has it. Extend this to the whole population and you have a world in which

50 percent of the men who don't have the boy-producing gene come home to reproduce, but 80 percent of the men who have it are still alive. In the next generation, therefore, there will be more boys than girls, and the sex ratio is once again more or less equalized. The daughters, who have not been sent into battle, are much more likely to survive, but since they don't carry the gene, they are as likely to have sons as daughters.

This oversimplifies things a bit, because there are other forces at work in maintaining the sex ratio. For example, if there are, for whatever reason, too many men around, there won't be enough women for all the men, and a higher percentage of women will be mothers than men will be fathers. So a man who is likely to produce more daughters has the advantage in the following generation—he's likely to have more grandchildren, and those grandchildren are likely to be girls. Sex ratio restored.

In China, because of the one-child-per-family rule, and because of a preference for male children, there are more boys than girls being born right now, putting the population's sex ratio out of balance. This can't last. As women become scarcer, a higher percentage of women than men will have offspring. Fathers with a genetic propensity to produce girls will regain the advantage, because they will be the ones more likely to have grandchildren.

Another wrinkle: slightly more boys than girls are born under any circumstances, about 103 boys for every 100 girls. But as we saw, at every age, more men than women die. This, too, contributes to restoring the balance.

Don't Blame Breast-feeding

Some doctors specialize in childhood cancers, others specialize in drooping breasts. Hey, it's a big wide medical world out there. Anyway, some drooping-breast specialists have discovered that it's not breast-feeding that makes breasts deflate.

A group of plastic surgeons reviewed the charts of ninety-three patients who had come to them for cosmetic breast surgery to see why these women's breasts weren't all they wanted them to be. (The article doesn't say who funded the research.) All of the patients had had babies, and 58 percent of them had breast-fed. The surgeons rated each woman's degree of breast droop based on photos taken before the operations, then compared the ratings to see whether it was breast-feeding that had caused the drooping. It wasn't, even

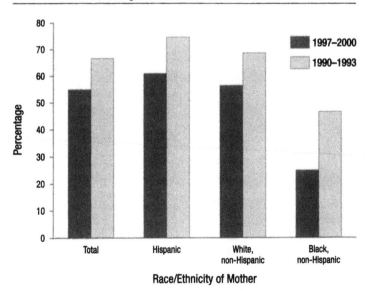

Percentage of Babies Who Were Breast-fed

though half of the patients claimed that their breast problems started after their pregnancies.

The study did find that certain things do lead to droopy breasts, including a higher number of pregnancies, a higher body mass index, and a history of smoking. The most significant factor, however, was pre-pregnancy bra cup size.

Breast-feeding is unquestionably the best way to feed infants in their first few months of life. Many women believe that breast-feeding will change the appearance of their breasts—in fact, in published reports, this fear is one of the major reasons women give for refusing to breast-feed. There may be good reasons not to breast-feed, but because you think it will make your breasts look bad is not one of them.

4

BEDSIDE MANNER

*Doctors cut, burn, and torture the
sick, and then demand of them an
undeserved fee for such services.*

—HERACLITUS OF EPHESUS (C. 540–480 BC)

How Valium (and Every Other Drug) Got Its Name

ALL DRUGS HAVE AT LEAST THREE NAMES. THE CHEMICAL
name specifies the molecular structure of the substance,
and only researchers use it. Doctors and pharmacists may
use the generic name, an abbreviation derived from the chemical name. And, like the rest of us, they'll also use the brand
name that the drug company has pounded into our heads with
TV commercials. Even a doctor or a pharmacist talking about
a common anxiety medication is not going to say "take a 7-
chloro-1-methyl-5-phenyl-3H-1,4-benzodiazepin-2-one"
when he or she can prescribe the generic diazepam, or, even
easier, just use the familiar brand name, Valium.

The chemical name is used when the drug is being

developed by researchers. When they're ready to start testing their invention to see if it works, the pharmaceutical company invents a shorter name as a generic, and submits it to a board called the United States Adopted Names Council (USANC), an organization cosponsored by the American Medical Association, the American Pharmacists Association, and the United States Pharmacopeia (they're the "USP" on drug labels). These are three private member organizations consisting of doctors, pharmacists, and scientists.

The USANC has its rules. The name has to be short and easy to pronounce. It can't imply efficacy or application to any particular body part. And it should be as different from other drug names as possible. After they're done approving the name, it's sent to the World Health Organization for final approval. When that is granted, the drug company can start testing the drug in animals to see if it's safe and effective.

In the case of Valium, it's pretty clear that the pharmaceutical company Hoffmann–La Roche selected "diazepam" for the similarity to one part of the chemical name. Drugs in the same class as diazepam, a benzodiazepine, are given similar-sounding generic names—alprazolam, lorazepam, and triazolam are all benzodiazepines. So are clonazepam, flurazepam, temazepam . . . but don't get us started.

It works the same way for other classes of drugs. If a drug has "barb" somewhere in the generic name, it's a barbiturate, like phenobarbital, amobarbital, or allobarbital; the "cillin" in amoxicillin, cloxacillin, ampicillin, or dicloxacillin indicates a drug from the penicillin class. Doxycycline, clomocycline, and minocycline are antibiotics of the tetracycline class, and fluoxetine, fluvoxamine, paroxetine, and others are SSRI antidepressants. The cancer drugs alemtuzumab, rituximab, and cetuximab end that way because "mab" stands for "monoclonal antibody." This system is useful, because it gives doctors and pharmacists a hint as to the class of a given drug and a quick idea of its indications and side effects.

But the drug company invents another name, too, one that is its own, and is used for the duration of the drug's patent, usually seventeen years. This is the one used in advertising, and therefore the one most consumers use when they buy the stuff. And so you have the brand name Valium, and lots of others. How a company comes up with a brand name involves all the tools of marketing plus many associated legal considerations.

Some letters look good in print, or seem kind of scientific, or powerful and effective—*X* and *Z* are special favorites, of which Xanax, Celebrex, Zyban, and Clarinex all take advantage. If you have a product you want to aim at women, adding "fem" in there somewhere seems like a good idea. Sarafem is just Prozac, but if you want to sell it to women with PMS, why not change the name? Sometimes the explanation is more prosaic—Lipitor, for example, one of the best-selling drugs of all time, takes the "lip" from "lipid regulator," which is what the drug is, and the "tor" from atorvastatin, the generic name. James L. Dettore, president of the Brand Institute, a branding company, was quoted as saying that Levitra, an erectile dysfunction drug, takes its name from "elevate," but it also sounds "European, elegant, with premium connotations." The "vit" looks like "vital," which is certainly a plus, and the "Le" part sure sounds French—French in a good way, of course: sophisticated and worldly.

Picking a name is not a casual exercise, and consultations with outside experts—lawyers and other varieties—can cost drug companies hundreds of thousands of dollars. The legal aspects of the trademark process are a particular

preoccupation. There are millions of trademarks, and infring-
ing one of them can lead to expensive lawsuits. Brand names
can be registered with the U.S. Patent and Trademark Office.
There's also a European patent and trademark office, and
names that are going to be used internationally can be registered there as well. Many drugs have multiple brand names
for marketing them in countries around the world.

What's Inside an Ambulance?

Exact requirements vary by state and agency, but this is the
equipment required by the New York State Emergency Medical Services for ambulance vehicles.

1 wheeled ambulance cot
1 stair chair or equivalent
1 patient-carrying device (stretcher, scoop, etc.), with 2 patient
    restraints on each device
2 crash-resistant securing devices for 2 patient-carrying de-
    vices
1 adult bag valve mask, with 2 different sizes of adult clear,
    air-cushion-type masks
1 pediatric bag valve mask, with clear face masks in newborn,
    infant, and child sizes
1 airway, oral, in 4 adult sizes (e.g., 80, 90, 100, 120 mm)
2 airways, oral, in 3 pediatric sizes (e.g., neonate, infant, child)
Oxygen, portable, "D"-size cylinders minimum, 2000 psi mini-
    mum pressure among cylinders, 15 lpm gauge, all gauges in-
    tact, with valid hydrostatic test date
Oxygen, on-board, 1200 liter, 500 psi minimum, 50 psi pres-

sure reducer, 2–15 lpm flow meters with simultaneous flow, with valid hydrostatic test date

4 non-rebreather oxygen masks, adult

2 non-rebreather oxygen masks, pediatric

4 nasal cannulae, oxygen, adult

2 nasal cannulae, oxygen, pediatric

1 suction, portable, 300 mmHg (if unit operates from vehicle electrical system, it can meet requirement of installed suction)

1 suction, installed, adjustable, vacuum or electric, 300 mmHg

2 suction catheters, rigid, plastic, yankauer type

2 suction catheters, flexible, sterile, 5, 8, 10 French sizing

2 suction devices, pediatric, bulb syringe or equivalent

1 spineboard, full-sized, 6'×16", with straps, nonporous coating

1 short spineboard or equivalent device, with straps

1 traction splint, including ankle hitch, mechanical tensioning device, ratchet, and slings

2 padded board splints, long, 4½'×3"

2 padded board splints, medium, 3'×3" or equivalent

2 padded board splints, short, 15"×3"

1 set extrication collars, large, medium, small, and pediatric or one adjustable adult and one pediatric

1 head immobilization device

24 dressings, gauze, sterile, 4"×4"

3 rolls tape, adhesive, 2 different sizes

10 rolls bandage, gauze, conforming, 2 different sizes

2 dressings, trauma, sterile, 10"×30" minimum

10 dressings, sterile, 5"×9"

1 pair scissors, bandage

2 burn sheets, sterile, bed sized

6 bandages, triangular
1 liter saline, sterile, within expiration date
1 dressing, occlusive, sterile
1 childbirth kit with sterile supplies
4 sheets, linen, including on cot
2 pillows
2 pillowcases
2 blankets
4 towels, cloth
1 box tissues, facial
2 emesis containers
1 blood pressure cuff, adult
1 blood pressure cuff, child (may be a set combined with adult)
1 blood pressure cuff, infant
1 stethoscope, adult
1 stethoscope, pediatric
1 case, carrying (jump kit)
4 cold packs
1 urinal, male
1 bedpan
2 eye protections for infection control (e.g., goggles, shield)
2 masks, infection control type
2 pr disposable gloves, rubber or plastic
1 glucose, liquid, or equivalent
6 sanitary napkins
1 flashlight (for patient assessment)
1 swaddler, infant
1 humidifier set with sterile water, disposable
6 flares or 3 reflective triangles
1 fire extinguisher, 10BC rating

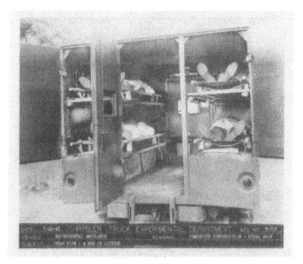

This World War II training ambulance does not meet the New York State requirements.

1 radio, 2-way or equivalent
1 lantern, battery operated (scene or interior lighting)

An ambulance must also have:

Valid Department of Motor Vehicles registration and inspection
Valid Department of Health inspection
Tires, exhaust, glass, lights, mechanical condition must be clean and sanitary, in good working order, and maintained per manufacturer's specifications
Agency name on 3 sides
Department of Health logo on 3 sides
Equipment secured, clean and sanitary, in good working order per manufacturer's specifications

Seat belts for driver, front passenger, all rear seats, and squad
bench
Heater and air-conditioning, operable
All equipment on board operable by EMT
Drugs locked in a cabinet

Afternoon Golf?

Golf isn't the only sport of choice for the athletically and med-
ically gifted. All these doctors were also splendid athletes.

Runner's high. On May 6, 1954, Roger Bannister (b. 1929) ran
a mile in 3 minutes 59.4 seconds, the first time that anyone
had run a mile in under four minutes. The performance is still
inspiring even though we know that today milers routinely post
times under 3:50 and then immediately carry on a perfectly calm
interview with the TV announcer, the only apparent effect of
the effort some slight panting that interferes with their re-
sponses.

The race was set up specifically for Bannister to try to break
the record. The weather in Oxford, England, was pretty bad—
crosswinds in gusts up to twenty-five miles an hour—and Bannister almost called the whole thing off. There were two
"rabbits" to set the pace for him, Chris Brasher and Chris
Chataway. Brasher took the lead at the start, and when he began to tire Chataway took over, leading at the start of the bell
lap. About two hundred yards from the finish, Bannister went
into his kick.

The track's announcer that day was Norris McWhirter,
later the founding editor of the *Guinness Book of Records.*

George Sheehan (1918–1993) was not only a runner but a

best-selling author. His book *Running and Being* and seven others made him (a) rich and (b) the priest-guru-philosopher king of running. He managed to turn ordinary physical exercise into an act of spiritual affirmation—no kidding. *New York Times* sports columnist Robert Lipsyte said of him: "George's mind always outran us. More than anyone, he widened running's moral purpose, which was not to live longer but to live better, to have more energy and self-worth and clarity for all the more important things in life." All this from putting on a pair of flimsy nylon shorts and running around in circles! If only we'd known.

Sheehan had also been an avid tennis player. According to some sources, he punched a wall in a fit of temper when a patient awakened him and hurt his hand so that he could no longer play tennis—which seems like a not terribly spiritual act for such a spiritual guy. Anyway, that's when the running started.

Sheehan gave up his medical practice in the early 1980s to devote himself full-time to writing and speaking about running. He died of prostate cancer, and his last book, *Going the Distance*, was published posthumously.

Iced up. Tenley Albright (b. 1935) was the first American woman to win an Olympic gold medal in figure skating. Her international skating career started in 1952, at the age of nineteen, when she won the U.S. singles championship—a feat she repeated for the next four years. She started college at Radcliffe in 1953, competing while going to school, and as a member of the U.S. Olympic team she won the gold at Cortina, Italy, in the 1956 Winter Games. She retired from competitive skating, finished up at Radcliffe, and graduated from Harvard Medical School in 1961, following her father into surgery.

Debi Thomas (b. 1967) won the world championship in figure skating in 1986, and the U.S. championship in 1986 and 1988. In the 1988 Olympics she won a bronze medal, and afterward spent several years performing in ice shows.

Thomas went to Stanford as an undergraduate and to Northwestern for medical school. She's a surgeon now in California, with a specialty in knee, hip, and other joint replacement. It's hard to say how many California surgeons employ a management company and have a professionally designed Web site that features press releases, photographs, flattering magazine clippings, and movies, and on top of that offers—free, if you send in a self-addressed stamped envelope!—autographed photographs of the doctor in 5" × 7" or 8" × 10" format. But Thomas is one of them.

It's very hard to win an Olympic gold medal, and presumably five times as hard to win five. But that is what Eric Heiden (b. 1958) did at the 1980 Winter Olympics in Lake Placid, New York. When he quit skating, he became a bicyclist, but his cycling career ended with a bang: in 1986, a member of the first American team in the Tour de France, he fell in the eighteenth stage, knocking himself out and ending his cycling career.

Heiden graduated from medical school at Stanford in 1991, became an orthopedic surgeon, and now practices in Davis, California. His wife, Karen, is also a surgeon.

Breakfast is the most important meal. Richard Besdine (b. 1940) is a professor of medicine at Brown University, specializing in geriatrics, and although his curriculum vitae says that he graduated from the University of Pennsylvania Medical School in 1965 and lists his more than ninety professional publications, it doesn't mention the fact that he is a champion squash player, still playing and winning tournaments in the sixty-five-and-over age group. He won the Massachusetts state championship in 1979, the Hartford Open in 1986, and a half dozen other tournaments here and there. He plays squash every day but, in the usual pattern for champion squash players, his face will never appear on the front of the Wheaties box, unless he orders a personalized version himself (available online for $32.95, plus additional charges for extra options).

House of Ruth calls. Cardiologist Bobby Brown (b. 1924) played eight seasons, 1946 to 1954 (with a year off for military service in 1953), for the New York Yankees. He was a utility infielder, mostly at third base, and retired with a batting average of .279.

But that was only one of his careers. It is almost certainly not true that Yogi Berra saw him reading a medical text, tossed aside the comic book he was reading, and asked Brown how his book came out, but of course a lot of stories about Yogi are probably not true, and no one really cares. A graduate of Stanford, Brown went to medical school at Tulane after his retirement from baseball, and practiced cardiology in the Dallas area through the early 1980s. That's when his third career began: he was appointed president of the American League in 1984, a post he served in for the next ten years.

We have no idea about his skills as a dentist, but Jim Lonborg (b. 1942) was a very good right-handed pitcher during his fifteen years in the big leagues. Probably his best years were with the Boston Red Sox in the 1960s. In 1967, the year the Sox finally won a pennant, he had a 22–9 won-lost record

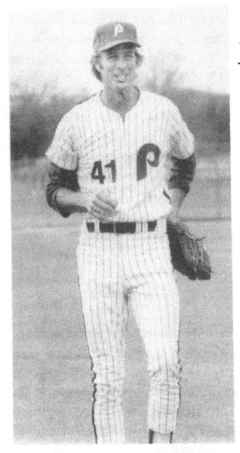

As #41 for the Phillies, Jim Lonborg didn't make it into sitcom history.

and an earned run average of 3.16. He was durable, too. Nine years later, now playing with the Phillies, he went 18–10 with a 3.08 e.r.a. He went to Tufts University Dental School, and has since practiced dentistry in Massachusetts.

In the 1980s sitcom *Cheers*, there's a photo of the bar's retired baseball player owner, Sam (played by Ted Danson), that hangs in the bar. It's actually a picture of Lonborg, who wore #16—Sam's number in the show.

And yes, golf. Cary Middlecoff (1921–1998) won the U.S. Open in 1949 and 1956 and the Masters in 1955, and was a regular winner in smaller events. But he was a dentist before he became a professional golfer, having graduated from dental school in 1944 and served as an army dentist during World War II.

Middlecoff was notorious for his slow play. In a play-off at the 1957 Open, his opponent Dick Mayer showed up with a camp stool, not so subtly commenting on Middlecoff's tendency to become a human rain delay. Middlecoff lost the playoff, shooting a miserable 79. But he is reputed to have said, "I always told myself that it didn't matter if I made it or missed it. My wife would still love me, and I'd still have steak for dinner."

Why Is It Called a Charley (or Charlie) Horse?

Wait a second. This isn't a book about word origins. So before we get into why it's called a charley horse, let's discuss exactly what a charley horse *is*. To some it apparently means a leg cramp. To others it's a sprained tendon or a muscle injury. Usually it's used to mean an injury to the quadriceps muscle of the leg. To make that official, the *Journal of the American Medical Association* published an article on November 30, 1946, in which it was defined as "an injury to a muscle, usually the quadriceps femoris." So let's call it a minor, somewhat painful, mildly debilitating injury, usually to the leg.

Apparently the first time it actually appeared in a general dictionary was in 1909, or so says an etymologist named H. B. Woolf in an article published in *American Speech* in 1973. Woolf describes an inquiry about the term from a dictionary editor to H. L. Mencken, who declined to answer but suggested that members of the old Baltimore Orioles team might "throw light on the matter," but that "they are now all angels" and therefore unavailable for comment. The guy did find a surviving Oriole, a fellow named Bill Clarke. Clarke said that there had been a left-handed pitcher on the team named Charley Esper, who had bad feet, pulled muscles a lot, and sometimes walked out to the mound with a limp. Clarke was pretty sure that Esper's teammates started calling him Charley Horse.

But pretty sure wasn't sure enough. In fact, the admirably persistent David Shulman wrote an article about it in the journal *American Speech* in 1949, arguing that the term appeared in a book called *Play Ball* by M. J. Kelley, published in 1888, before Esper started playing. So the Esper story doesn't work.

Someone suggested that the Sioux City team in the Western League had a horse named Charley who was used to drag the diamond, and he put his feet up and down so gingerly that when a player with a sore muscle went out onto the field, they'd say, "Here comes Charley." Others mentioned other horses, or other ballplayers, who were supposed to have either inspired or coined the term. But in the end it remains a mystery.

You Still Can't Read Their Writing

These twelve doctors (and a dentist) didn't let the professional reputation for bad penmanship get in the way of their literary aspirations:

François Rabelais (c. 1483–1553), the French humanist, wrote the five satirical novels called *The Life of Gargantua and Pantagruel* and practiced medicine throughout his life.

Tobias Smollett (1721–1771) is generally considered the first Scottish novelist. He wrote the picaresque adventures

Roderick Random, Peregrine Pickle, and *Humphrey Clinker.* Smollett also spent several years as a naval surgeon.

Friedrich von Schiller (1759–1805) is the author of the plays *The Robbers, Mary Stuart, The Maid of Orleans,* and *Don Carlos.* This Sturm und Drang movement poet, essayist, and dramatist became a regimental surgeon after medical school but practiced only for a few years. In 2008, the German newsweekly *Der Spiegel* reported that a DNA test had discovered that the skull in Schiller's coffin was not his own.

Oliver Wendell Holmes Sr. (1809–1894), the American poet and essayist, is perhaps most famous for *The Autocrat of the Breakfast-Table.* But he's also the author of *The Contagiousness of Puerperal Fever,* which concluded, contrary to medical belief at the time, that the disease was carried from patient to patient by doctors. Holmes taught medicine at Harvard for more than thirty years. He is said to be the inspiration for the name of Sherlock Holmes, the fictional detective created by another doctor.

Arthur Conan Doyle (1859–1930) is the other doctor. As the story goes, he knew of an actual "consulting detective" named Wendel Scherer, whose name Doyle converted to Sherlock, with Oliver Wendell Holmes as his second inspiration. Sherlock Holmes's friend and partner, Watson, is of course a doctor, and the stories are filled with medical terms and references to diseases, drugs, medical schools, and medical journals. They also contain fictional counterparts of some of Doyle's real patients. Doyle continued practicing medicine after he published the Sherlock Holmes stories, and he served as a field doctor during the Boer War.

Anton Chekhov (1860–1904) wrote *The Cherry Orchard, The Sea-Gull, Three Sisters,* and *Uncle Vanya,* among many other plays and hundreds of short stories. He practiced

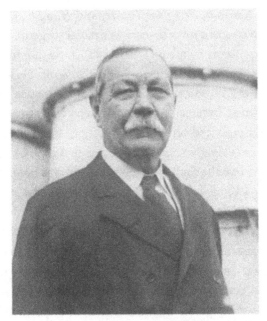

*Arthur Conan Doyle, MD, claimed that not a single
patient visited his ophthalmology practice in Vienna.
This, presumably, gave him plenty of time to write.*

medicine all his life. He struggled with tuberculosis for many
years (his brother Nicolai succumbed to the disease in 1889),
and he died at a spa in Badenweiler, Germany.

Somerset Maugham (1874–1965) served as a doctor for a
short time after medical school but quickly abandoned medicine for writing, his real passion. This Englishman is the author of *Of Human Bondage*, *The Razor's Edge*, *The Moon and
Sixpence*, *Cakes and Ale*, and many other novels, plays, and
film scripts.

Mikhail Bulgakov (1891–1940), the Russian novelist, play-
wright, and short story writer, is most known for his retelling
of the Faust legend, *The Master and Margarita*. He also wrote

a memoir of his life as a rural doctor, *A Country Doctor's Notebook*. He died from nephrosclerosis, a genetic kidney disorder.

William Carlos Williams (1883–1963) won a posthumous Pulitzer Prize for *Pictures from Brueghel and Other Poems*. How this full-time pediatrician found time to write novels, essays, short stories, prizewinning poetry, and an autobiography is a mystery, if not a medical one.

Walker Percy (1916–1990) won the National Book Award for his first novel, *The Moviegoer*. He contracted tuberculosis as an intern at Bellevue Hospital in New York, and spent the next few years recuperating at a sanatorium. After recovering, he took up writing full-time and never practiced medicine again. He published five other novels and many works of nonfiction.

Robin Cook (b. 1940) is the author of more than two dozen thrillers, almost all of which have medicine as a background—including *Contagion*, *Toxin*, *Vector*, and *Seizure*.

Michael Crichton (1942–2008) wrote more than twenty novels, several films and television programs, and several works of nonfiction, many with medical themes. He graduated from Harvard Medical School (he supported himself as a student by writing thrillers under a pseudonym), but never actually practiced medicine because of the success of his first book published under his own name, *The Andromeda Strain*.

Zane Grey (1872–1939) is the one dentist in our list. He was also a minor league baseball player, but that was before he practiced dentistry and wrote about five dozen cowboy novels.

Lost in Prescription

Rx is the usual abbreviation for "prescription," but its origin is unclear. Some believe that it comes from the Latin *recipere*, meaning "to take." Others say it has an Egyptian origin. Among themselves, doctors often use abbreviations that look a lot like Rx—sx for signs or symptoms, dx for diagnosis, tx for treatment, hx for history.

In any case, here's what the abbreviations on an Rx mean, in alphabetical order:

ac	(ante cibum): before meals
bid	(bis in die): twice a day
gt	(gutta): drop
hs	(hora somni): at bedtime
od	(oculus dexter): right eye
os	(oculus sinister): left eye
pc	(post cibum): after meals
po	(per os): by mouth
prn	(pro re nata): as needed
q3h	(quaque 3 hora): every 3 hours
qd	(quaque die): every day
qid	(quater in die): 4 times a day
sig	(signa): write
tid	(ter in die): 3 times a day

5

LAB RAT

*I am convinced that of all quackeries,
the physician's is the grotesquest & the
silliest. And they know they are shams
& humbugs. They have taken the place
of those augurs who couldn't look each
other in the face without laughing.*

—MARK TWAIN (1835–1910)

The Routine Blood Test

ABLOOD TEST IS EASY: THE NURSE JUST STICKS YOU, COL-lects some blood, and sends it off to the lab. And a blood test can produce some useful information. Usually if there's something that comes back looking suspicious, that isn't the end of the story—the doctor then has to figure out *why* there's an abnormal test result.

Here are the usual tests you get at the average annual physical exam:

Liver function tests. The liver is the body's protein factory and is essential in removing toxins. Tests check levels of the enzymes alanine aminotransferase (ALT), aspartate aminotransferase (AST) (found in many organs in addition to the liver), and alkaline phosphatase (also found in many organs); direct and indirect bilirubin, which is excreted in bile and causes the distinct yellow hue of bruises and jaundice; and albumin, a protein synthesized by the liver. There's also a measure of prothrombin time, which is a test of your blood clotting. Most blood-clotting factors are made in the liver, so an irregular result might point to a reason for otherwise unexplained bleeding.

Kidney function tests. The kidneys filter waste matter and keep the proper electrolyte balance in the body. Blood urea nitrogen (BUN) levels show whether toxic products are being properly eliminated from your body. Creatinine levels indicate whether your electrolytes are in balance, while serum electrolytes—sodium bicarbonate, potassium, calcium, magnesium—look at which electrolytes are low or high. Doctors also look at uric acid, a toxin that usually exits the body in urine, as the name suggests.

Complete blood count. The volume of red blood cells tells whether you're anemic and whether the blood is carrying oxygen properly; the volume of white blood cells can indicate infection, allergy, or inflammation. Platelet count provides another measure of blood clotting.

Cholesterol and lipid tests. Total cholesterol level—which everyone these days knows should be under 200—is a combination of several different types of cholesterol, some of which cause atherosclerosis (the ominous buildup of plaque in your arteries) and some of which fight against the types that cause atherosclerosis. Low density lipoproteins (LDL) are "bad" cholesterol; the more of them, the greater your risk for heart disease. High density lipoproteins (HDL) are "good" cholesterol, which helps the body rid itself of bad cholesterol. Very low density lipoproteins (VLDL) are yet another kind of bad cholesterol—as though there wasn't enough to worry about—and triglycerides, a type of fat, should be watched, too.

Thyroid function tests. Thyrotropin-releasing hormone (TRH) is produced by the hypothalamus. This substance causes your pituitary gland to release thyroid-stimulating hormone (TSH), which makes your thyroid release two more hormones, triiodothyronine (T3) and thyroxine (T4). All these tests together determine if your thyroid is working properly.

We suggest you not try these at home.

Of Mice and Men

The evolutionary lineages of man and mouse diverged about 96 million years ago, but the close relationship of the two species has persisted. The common house mouse was first an agricultural pest, then a pet, and now the most common and useful organism for understanding human biology: we use about 25 million each year in scientific experiments. Dogs are nice, but there's really no contest: mice are man's best friend.

We are very like mice in our bodily organs and the structure of our tissue, and we suffer from many of the same diseases. Both the human and mouse genomes have been sequenced and mapped—we know what and where the genes

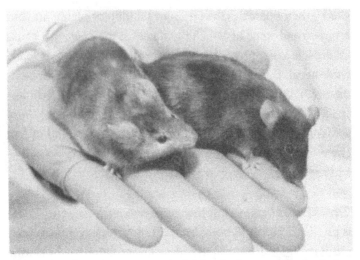

What a knockout: the mouse on the left has had a gene affecting hair growth knocked out; the one on the right is normal.

are—and, gee, *Homo sapiens* shares 95 percent of its genetic makeup with *Mus musculus*. We also share large linkage groups—genes that are known to be transmitted together—and their order along the chromosomes.

Because gene mapping and sequencing technologies are so good, geneticists are finding genes that affect or control many human diseases and behaviors. Practically every day, there is news of the discovery of a gene that affects this or that human malady. But finding a gene for a disease is a far cry from finding a cause or a treatment. We have a mapped genome, but we don't have a functional guide that tells us what the genes actually *do*. This is where the so-called knockout mouse comes in.

We have learned to insert a gene at a precise location in the mouse genome. This means that scientists can inject an inactive gene in a fertilized embryo that replaces a particular gene of interest. Then a line of mice can be bred that lack that gene. By experimenting with these mice, the effect of the gene can be determined.

There are several companies that sell knockout mice. One of the largest is the Jackson Laboratory in Bar Harbor, Maine. It has mice that are genetically obese, mice that are prone to skin rashes or asthma or epileptic seizures, mice that almost always become diabetic, mice that have a high incidence of sarcomas that resemble Hodgkin's disease. There are hybrids that are very robust and good as hosts for transplanted tumors. You can buy mice that have no hair, or mice that lose their hair in patches. Or you can buy one of several different strains that are subject to age-related hearing loss—they start to become deaf before they're three months old. There are mice that get arthritis, lupus, intestinal cancer, cardiovascular disease, retinal degeneration, high cholesterol, leukemia, abnormal breathing, liver disease, or severe immune deficiency—take your pick. Jackson has recently developed a mouse that is extremely diabetic, underweight, and hungry all the time, urinates copiously, and has severe kidney, skeletal, and testicular defects. It even has a strain that's good for producing more transgenic mice because they have fertilized eggs that are ideal for injecting with foreign DNA.

Making a knockout mouse is very expensive—it can cost anywhere from $3,000 to $30,000 to produce a custom model. Depending on the strain and the age—older ones cost more—you can pay between $20 and more than $200 for a single mouse. Sometimes females are slightly more expensive than males. Jackson also maintains large colonies of mice that occasionally produce spontaneous mutations, and when it has a lot of them, it sells them for 20 percent off—"while supplies last."

The Trouble with Twins

More than a century ago, Darwin's cousin Sir Francis Galton and other scientists realized that fraternal and identical twins present a natural experiment in genetics. (Galton also coined the term "eugenics" and came up with a method for analyzing fingerprints.) Since identical twins share the same genes, and fraternal twins share only 50 percent of theirs, the characteristics that match in identical, but not in fraternal, twins can be attributed to genes and not environment.

Moreover, if you studied the differences between identical twins raised in different families—people with the exact same genetic makeup but different environments—you could an-

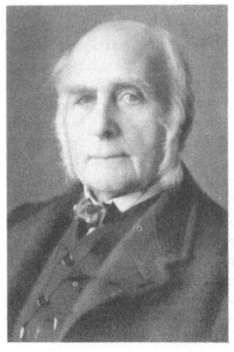

Sir Francis Galton, Darwin's cousin, was obsessed with heredity.

swer even more questions about which traits or behaviors were caused by nature and which by nurture. It was a neat idea, and there are many studies comparing identical and fraternal twins, or identical twins raised apart.

This is the classical view of twin studies, which would be nice if it really worked. But it probably doesn't, because there are some serious complications.

If people choose mates in part because they are genetically similar to them, then fraternal twins would share more than 50 percent of their genes. Identical twins, even those raised together, may have very different environments, beginning with their position in the womb and carrying on throughout their lives. Identical twins may be treated by parents and others more similarly than fraternal twins, making their environments more alike than that of fraternals. Interactions between genes and environment may determine physical and psychological traits, making the contribution of each difficult to ascertain.

Geneticists have also figured out that two individuals may have the same genes, but environment can make certain genes active—turn them on, so to speak—while others remain dormant. These "turned on" genes, it appears, can even be inherited. Identical twins, in short, are not as identical as we once thought.

The Truth About Coffee

Studies of human nutrition are notoriously difficult to carry out. You can ask people what they eat, and you can get them to keep diaries. But the data you get are not likely to be accurate. Most people can hardly remember what they ate for breakfast, never mind offering an accurate account of what they habitually eat over long periods of time. Also, people lie about some things, especially alcohol—they often say they drink less than they really do. Of course, you could hospitalize people and experimentally feed them only certain kinds of food. But that's very expensive, and it's difficult to get people to agree to be hospitalized and put on an experimental diet, and you can't keep people hospitalized long enough to see the effects of a diet over time. Moreover, even if a researcher got the money to set up such a study, the dropout rate would likely be high.

But coffee is different. Everyone knows how much coffee they drink, and they don't lie about it. And people drink the same amount of coffee every day for long periods of time. If you're a fifty-year-old coffee drinker, chances are you've drunk almost exactly the same amount of coffee every day for the past twenty-five years or more. That's good data—a researcher knows exactly how much you've drunk; you've drunk a lot, so he or she can see some effects; and you've done it for long periods of time. All that makes for very good information from which accurate conclusions can be drawn. Which is why people who study nutrition like to study coffee.

Can I Donate Blood?

According to the Red Cross, you can donate blood if you're healthy, at least seventeen years old (or sixteen, in some locales), and you weigh at least 110 pounds. By "healthy," it means that you feel well and can perform normal, everyday activities—including getting yourself to the blood drive. It will take about two months to replace the blood you part with, so you have to wait eight weeks before donating again. You normally donate about a pint each time.

Double red cell donation is an automated process in which you can donate two units of blood in one session by giving just red blood cells instead of red cells, plasma, and platelets. The red blood cells are in the most demand. The process uses a smaller needle than regular donation, and that may be more comfortable for you, too.

But to do it, you have to meet some special requirements. The U.S. Food and Drug Administration requires that men be at least 5 feet 1 inch tall and weigh 130 pounds, and—perhaps surprisingly—that women be at least 5 feet 5 inches and weigh 150. The qualifications are based on blood volume, and men have greater blood volume than women for the same size body. Both men and women need a hematocrit reading of at least 40—that is, 40 percent of your blood volume has to be red cells. You won't be able to donate blood again for four months, which is how long it will take to replenish your red blood cells.

You can also donate other blood components, such as platelets or plasma, rather than whole blood.

You can't donate blood if you have any of a number of diseases and disorders: hepatitis, AIDS, certain types of cancer, heart disease, severe asthma, malaria, bleeding disorders, or low blood pressure. Being pregnant, having had recent surgery, or using certain drugs will also get you off the hook. If you have diabetes or hypertension, you can still donate, but you have to be under treatment and the disease has to be under control.

There are a number of other ways you can be disqualified. For example, you can't give blood if you've traveled in the last year to a country where malaria is found. And if you've lived in such a country, you can't give blood until you've stopped living there for three years. This means that if you've traveled recently to Mexico, Haiti, the Dominican Republic, or almost anywhere in South America, Africa, or Asia, you aren't eligible to donate blood. Travel in sub-Saharan Africa causes the greatest risk, but on its Web site the CDC notes, in red letters, "If you are traveling outside of the United States, Canada, and Western Europe, you may be at risk for malaria."

People are sometimes rejected because their iron levels are too low, but this is often a temporary problem, and you can try again later.

You can donate your own blood if you're having surgery, a process called autologous donation. You do this about a month before your operation, and the hospital will store the blood for your use if you later need a transfusion. And you can donate blood for a specific friend or relative.

Donating blood is very safe. The transmission of disease—especially HIV and hepatitis, but other diseases as well—has historically been the greatest risk. But because present practice requires that any material that comes in contact with blood be used only once, and because both donors and blood are screened for infections, those risks have been reduced to near zero. You can feel light-headed or otherwise uncomfortable after donating blood, but the feeling goes away pretty quickly. The needle insertion can cause a bruise, but the risk of that is no greater than when you have blood taken for a blood test. Sometimes people faint because the volume of fluid in the body declines, causing a rapid decline in blood pressure. Almost no one has a serious bad reaction. One study looked at 194,000 donations and found only one donor with long-term problems.

6

BIOHAZARD!

Doctors is all swabs.

—ROBERT LOUIS STEVENSON (1850–1894)

How to Tell a Cold from the Flu

COLDS AND FLU SHARE MANY OF THE SAME SYMPTOMS, AND it can be difficult or impossible to tell the difference without laboratory tests to determine what kind of germ is causing the problem. In most cases, it doesn't matter which disease you have—it'll go away by itself anyway. In some cases, doctors might want to know, and they can find out, provided the test is done within the first few days after the symptoms start.

But there are ways to guess fairly reliably what is happening to you. A cold usually involves little more than a runny or stuffed-up nose and mild discomfort. In adults and older children, there's usually no fever. With a cold, you can get an irritated throat, but it's usually not red. You might get a headache, depending on which virus is causing the cold (there are about two hundred different species that can be involved), and you might get a cough or muscle aches. After a few days, nasal secretions become thicker, and sometimes yellow or green.

With a flu, you usually get a sudden fever, followed by body aches, tiredness, a dry cough, and a red throat. You feel sick all over. Sometimes there's dizziness or vomiting. Unlike cold viruses, which generally stay around the nose, flu viruses can go all over the respiratory tract, so you can wind up with lung and ear infections, too. The dry, hacking cough is probably the most characteristic symptom of the flu.

The World's Six Worst Infectious Diseases

You've heard a lot about strange infectious diseases like Ebola and Marburg virus—they make great copy—but they're actually quite rare. The diseases that really kill lots of people are fairly ordinary. In fact, there are six diseases—you've heard of all of them—that account for 90 percent of all deaths from infectious disease.

Pneumonia. Caused by many things, including the influenza virus, it generally kills between 10,000 and 40,000 Americans every flu season. But most of the deaths from pneumonia occur in developing countries and affect children particularly, with more than 3 million people dying each year.

HIV/AIDS. There are about 40 million people living with AIDS, and there are more than 4 million new HIV infections every year, including 40,000 a year in the United States. In 2006, 2.9 million people died of AIDS. More than 25 million have died of AIDS since 1981.

Diarrhea. This is really a group of diseases with a common deadly symptom. Two million children a year die from dehydration caused by diarrhea from cholera, dysentery, typhoid fever, rotavirus, and other diseases. Epidemics strike adults as well.

Tuberculosis. Once, this disease was thought to be under control. It has bounced back with a vengeance, killing 1.5 million people a year—not counting the one-third of AIDS deaths that are caused by TB. Two billion people—one-third of the world's population—have the disease in a latent form, an immense pool from which the disease can spread. According to the CDC, there were 12,898 cases of tuberculosis in the United States in 2008, the lowest since reporting began in 1953. The disease is widespread in sub-Saharan Africa, with the highest rates reported in Djibouti, Kenya, Namibia, Zambia, Zimbabwe, and South Africa. Perhaps the highest rate of all is in Swaziland, where the World Health Organization reports a rate of 469 infections per 100,000 people. The U.S. rate is about 2 per 100,000.

Malaria. Malaria comes from a bite of a female anopheles mosquito that got the malaria parasite when it bit an infected person. It's nasty, causing high fevers, convulsions, and breathing difficulties, and kills about a million people a year, mostly children, and mostly in sub-Saharan Africa. In the most severe type—cerebral malaria—a person can lapse into a coma and die within twenty-four hours. There are about 1,300 cases of malaria diagnosed in the United States every year, almost all of them in travelers returning from places where the disease is endemic. But there are two anopheles species that still live in the United States, and about five or six people get the disease without having left the country. Although malaria was

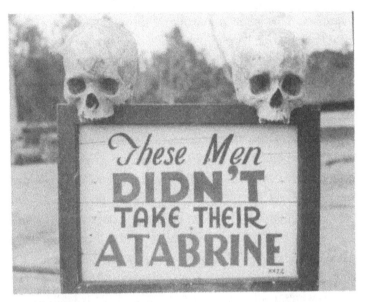

World War II enemy: malaria.

wiped out in the United States in the 1950s, the disease seems to be making a comeback.

Measles. Yes, measles. One of the most contagious diseases known, it killed about 242,000 children in 2006, mostly in developing countries. By some calculations, the measles virus, with its complications of pneumonia, diarrhea, and malnutrition, is responsible for more deaths than any other microbe. Happily, the measles vaccine has reduced the rate of infection by nearly half between 1999 and 2006, and the virus has almost disappeared in the United States.

Almost, but not quite. The largest outbreak in ten years occurred in the spring of 2008, sickening more than 120 people in fifteen states. Most of the cases were in children whose parents refused to vaccinate them for religious or other reasons.

Ten Diseases You Can Get from
Your Dog or Your Cat

The family pet causes several million infections every year, everything from minor rashes to life-threatening diseases. Usually these illnesses are not very serious. Every once in a while, they are.

Here are ten you can get from ordinary dogs and cats— and we don't even have to mention rabies, do we?

Toxoplasmosis. This is one of the most common pet-related diseases, caused by a protozoan, *Toxoplasma gondii.* The infection develops in cats and is excreted in their feces in the form of an oocyst that releases infectious spores. If you're not careful cleaning the litter box, you can pick it up on your hands. Gardening in soil that has feces in it is another route, and dogs can transmit it because they like to roll around in the stuff. It's not a serious illness in most people, but in rare cases it causes birth defects in the children of women exposed during the first trimester of pregnancy. It can also be a serious problem in people who are immunocompromised.

Toxocariasis. Toxocara is a roundworm that infects dogs and cats. Ingesting feces is the way to get it, and before you "poo-poo" the idea, this can happen to kids playing in sandboxes that animals have used as a toilet. It's usually not a serious infection, but sometimes the bugs can migrate to the liver or lungs, causing visceral larva migrans in about ten thousand Americans a year. This can lead to fever, abdominal pain, itchy skin, and wheezing—or, more seriously, inflammation of the heart or seizures. It usually goes away on its own, but it can be treated with any of a number of antiparasitic drugs.

Cutaneous larva migrans. Hookworm eggs in dog and cat feces hatch out, and the larvae can penetrate human skin. You can pick them up by walking around barefoot near feces, say, in your backyard. The larvae can't reproduce in humans, but they can crawl around under your skin, creating a rash as they travel. It itches, especially at night, and can be treated with albendazole and other antiworm drugs.

Plague. Yes, plague, the black death. The natural reservoir of this old favorite is wild rodents, and humans get infected through the bites of fleas that have fed on them, or through handling infected animals. Where plague is endemic, people have to be very careful to keep fleas away from their dogs and cats, because if the pets have fleas, so will the people who keep them, and if those fleas are infected with the plague bacterium, *Yersinia pestis*, they can transmit plague to humans.

The last time there was actually an epidemic in the United States was in Los Angeles in 1924 and 1925, but about fifteen cases are reported yearly. Most of them occur in the Southwest—northern New Mexico, northern Arizona, southern Colorado, and western Nevada—as well as California and southern Oregon. If your dog or cat has fleas and you live in an area where plague is endemic, there's a chance those fleas have been a bit promiscuous in their blood sucking, and you could catch the plague.

Plague causes lung damage and blood coagulation, and mortality is very high. You get a high fever, chills, cough, and breathing difficulty, and you may cough up blood. Without treatment, you'll probably die—the death rate is as high as 90 percent. That death toll goes down to about 15 percent if you are treated quickly with antibiotics.

Cat-scratch disease. Caused by a bacterium called *Bartonella henselae*, in humans this disease is usually transmitted by a scratch, lick, or bite from a cat that has been bitten by a carrier flea. While it used to be thought of mainly as a children's disease, about half of cases now occur in adults. You get a rash at the place where the infection started, and then an inflammation of the lymph nodes that goes away in a few weeks. It's not very dangerous in otherwise healthy people, but immunocompromised people can get seriously ill from it.

Lyme disease. Ticks of the genus Borrelia pick up the bacterium by feeding on infected deer, mice, squirrels, and other animals. Dogs are a vector—they bring in ticks from outside, and you can get the disease while removing them. That's how you can get Lyme disease without even going outside.

Most cases can be treated successfully with a few weeks of antibiotics, but sometimes even after treatment the symptoms can last for months or even years. About 60 percent of patients begin to have intermittent bouts of arthritis after a few months. A small minority of untreated patients get shooting pains or tingling in the hands or feet and memory and concentration problems. No one knows why symptoms persist, but some suspect that the person's immune system continues to respond after the infection has cleared.

MRSA. Methicillin-resistant *Staphylococcus aureus* (the bacterial infection that can, in extreme cases, lead to flesh-eating disease) is transmitted not only human to human, but also human to pet and pet to human. Dogs and cats can catch it from an infected person, and they can pass it back and forth. Dogs that visit health care facilities have been implicated in its transmission.

Pasteurella. A bacterial disease common in rabbits, cats, and dogs can also carry it, and you can get it by close contact—if the animal licks, bites, or scratches you. Kissing an infected animal is a good way to get it. It can in rare cases cause serious human illness, including pneumonia and peritonitis, an infection of the lining of the abdominal cavity.

Brucellosis. A dog disease that humans can catch—but rarely—it causes a fever that can progress to endocarditis, a serious infection of the heart. It's actually more commonly transmitted through consumption of unpasteurized dairy products or exposure to infected livestock.

Leptospirosis. This is one of the most common diseases people get from animals worldwide, but it's uncommon in the United States. Dogs are the main carriers, and you get it from contact with their urine or other body fluids—excluding saliva. Human infection resembles a mild flu and only rarely has serious complications.

Exotic and Deadly

For some people, dogs and cats just don't do it. So they keep frogs, toads, monkeys, rabbits, mice, rats, ferrets, hamsters, gerbils, prairie dogs, chinchillas, turtles, lizards, and iguanas. Sometimes they pick up a baby squirrel or chipmunk and try to raise it at home. Foxes, coyotes, wolves—there are people who will try to keep all of them, even if only temporarily, as pets. They're exotic. And they can also be dangerous, especially to children.

Many of these exotic pets can be found right here in the

United States, and still others are imported. In 2005, 87,991 mammals, including twenty-nine different species of rodents, were imported. So were 1.3 million reptiles, 203,000 fish, and 365,000 birds. And those are just the ones legally brought into the country. God only knows how many were illegally imported and what species they were. Some estimates value the trade in illegal exotic animals as high as $10 billion, which would mean that only the trade in illegal drugs and arms exceed it. This adds up to a flood of animals that can introduce pathological organisms, some of them quite novel and deadly.

Diseases that come from animals are not rare. In fact, in a list of 1,415 human pathogens put together by one group of scientists, 61 percent are known to come from animals. Among newly emerging infectious diseases, the percentage is even higher.

Tularemia. In 2002, wild-caught prairie dogs held in a Texas commercial facility caused an outbreak of tularemia in humans. The infected animals were distributed to pet stores in Texas, and some wound up as far away as the Czech Republic. Tularemia, sometimes called rabbit fever, is caused by a bacterium and can be transmitted in airborne form as well as by ticks, deerflies, and more petlike animals. It causes skin ulcers, swollen and painful lymph glands, muscle ache, headaches, joint pain, dry cough, and progressive weakness. Sometimes you get pneumonia from it—chest pain, difficulty breathing, bloody sputum. About two hundred cases a year are reported in the United States.

A very small number of bacteria—as few as ten of them—can cause the disease, and left untreated it can kill you. Two pieces of good news: it can be treated with antibiotics and you can't catch it from another person.

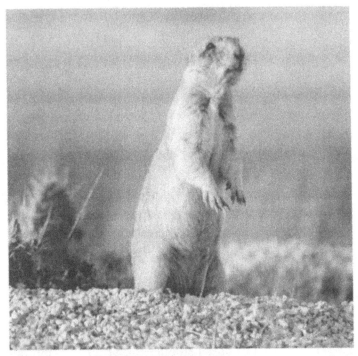

Beware the (potentially) dangerous prairie dogs of New Mexico.

Monkeypox. Prairie dogs were also responsible for the first cluster of human monkeypox cases in the United States in 2003. The suspicion is that the prairie dogs got sick after contact with various African rodents with the virus that had been imported as pets. The infections probably happened in a wholesale pet store—and we don't know where this pet store that sells prairie dogs and Gambian rats is located. Monkeypox gives you fever, headache, muscle ache, and swollen lymph nodes. You get a rash after a few days, which usually starts on the face and then spreads over the body. The rash grows into raised bumps filled with fluid. As they heal, they scab over and fall off. In Africa, the disease kills between 1 and 10 percent of the people who get infected, but there's better access to medical care in the United States and the chances of dying are considerably less. Epidemiologic studies have demonstrated that the most severe infections occur in children and in people who have not been vaccinated for smallpox.

Salmonellosis. Reptiles and amphibians are great for transmitting salmonellosis. It's usually not a serious illness—a couple of days of vomiting and diarrhea and you're done with it—but every once in a while it kills someone. Of course, you can get a salmonella infection from contaminated mayonnaise at a picnic or a piece of undercooked chicken, but 6 percent of all salmonella cases in the United States—74,000 cases a year—come from direct or indirect contact with reptiles or amphibians.

The first documented rodent-caused outbreak of salmonellosis occurred in 2004, when the disease was transmitted to humans by a hamster in South Carolina and a mouse in Minnesota. The CDC reported that fifteen patients in seven states were infected. Most of them were kids, and they had symptoms ranging from stomach cramps to fever to vomiting to bloody diarrhea. Six of them had to be hospitalized, but none of them died. Ominously, the strain of salmonella they had was resistant to five different antibiotics.

In 1998, a group of children attending a reptile exhibit caught salmonellosis. Animals kept in public settings where people have close contact with them—petting zoos, science exhibits, schools, community events, and so on—are great transmitters of disease. From 1991 through 2005, the CDC reported more than fifty-five outbreaks of illness involving animals in public settings. *E. coli* is commonly transmitted on visits to farms, petting zoos, livestock exhibits, and farm day camps.

Herpes B. Macaque monkeys are kept by some people, mostly illegally, and they're exhibited in public places by others, sometimes legally and sometimes not. Herpes B virus is endemic among them, and the virus has been transmitted to humans by bites, scratches, and splashes of infected material to human mucous membranes. The disease is a stone-cold killer: human infections often result in a fatal swelling of the brain called meningoencephalitis. These infections, to be sure, are infrequent, but people who survive them often have permanent neurological impairments. There's a drug, acyclovir, that seems to help, but it has not been widely used. The CDC reports that macaque species have escaped to establish free-ranging feral populations in Texas and Florida.

We make a special note that it's illegal to import these animals for anything other than scientific use or exhibit in legitimate zoos. It's also illegal to breed them or distribute them for any other purpose. You're not allowed to keep a macaque and then exhibit it from time to time and claim that that's legal. It isn't.

The Twenty-four Vaccine-Preventable Diseases

Some vaccines are given routinely to babies; most kids have to receive certain vaccines before they enroll in school. Some are only useful for people in certain jobs, or who travel to certain places, or who are of a certain age. Yet even with all of these vaccines, only one disease has been wiped out: smallpox.

Anthrax. For those who are exposed to large amounts of anthrax on the job or are at risk of getting attacked with a biological weapon. Since 2006, the U.S. Department of Defense has made receiving the anthrax vaccine mandatory for military personnel.

Cholera. Two types of oral vaccine are available for travelers to endemic areas, but the risk of cholera for travelers is low, and the vaccine is only partially effective. Still, some countries may at some times require it for entry.

Diphtheria. All kids should get this vaccine, starting at age five months. It's usually given along with the tetanus and pertussis (whooping cough) vaccines in a form called DTaP.

Haemophilius influenzae type b (Hib). All kids should get this vaccine, in a course of four doses starting when they are two months old. Most adults don't need it, unless they are immunocompromised or have other special health conditions.

Hepatitis A. All children should get this vaccine when they're one year old. Many adults should get it, too, including people who travel to countries with a high prevalence of the illness, or who live in areas of high prevalence. Gay men and people who have chronic liver disease are also encouraged to get it.

Hepatitis B. Everyone under age eighteen should be vaccinated, as should adults who have more than one sex partner in six months. Health care workers should get it, too, as should anyone who has contact with someone who has the disease.

Human papillomavirus (HPV). Approved in 2006, this vaccine is recommended for girls ages eleven and twelve, and can be given to girls as young as nine. It can prevent most genital warts and most cases of cervical cancer.

Influenza (flu). Children six months to nineteen years, pregnant women, people over age fifty, people of any age with certain medical conditions, people who live in nursing homes, and anyone who works with or lives with anyone at high risk for complications from the flu should all get the vaccine. That's a lot of people.

Japanese encephalitis. Only laboratory workers and people who travel in rural parts of Asia should be vaccinated for this disease. Not for kids under one year of age.

Meningococcal disease. This disease kills about two hundred people a year in spite of treatment with antibiotics. In December 2007, the vaccine was approved for children ages two to ten who are at increased risk for the disease, especially those who have HIV; the vaccine had previously been approved for people over age eleven. There are two kinds, both of which work well, but the new MCV4 may give longer-lasting protection than the older MPSV4. People with certain health conditions that affect the immune system should get it, too.

Measles. Given along with the vaccines for mumps and rubella—the MMR vaccine. All kids should get this, in two doses, starting at one year of age. And anyone eighteen or older born after 1956 should get it, too, unless they can show that they have had either the vaccine or the diseases.

Mumps. See above, under *Measles.*

Pertussis (whooping cough). See above, under *Diphtheria.*

Pneumococcal disease. You may never have heard of this one, but more than 230,000 people are infected with pneumococcal disease every year in the United States, not counting the 5 million kids who get ear infections from it. When it infects the lining of the brain, it is fatal in about one-third of cases. There are two vaccines, one called pneumococcal polysaccharide, or PPV23, the other called pneumococcal conjugate vaccine, or PCV7. PPV23 should be given to all adults over age sixty-five, and to anyone over two years old who has a condition or a medical regimen that lowers immunity. PCV7 should be given to children under two in four doses beginning at two months. Kids ages two to five should also get it if they have medical conditions that warrant it.

Polio. Developed by Jonas Salk in 1952, this vaccine may follow the historical landmark set by the smallpox shot: in 2007 only 1,310 cases of polio were reported around the world. All kids should get four doses starting at two months. Adults usually don't need it unless they're traveling to places where the disease is still common, or are health care or lab workers likely to come in contact with it.

Rabies. This neurological disease causing encephalitis can be transmitted by animal bite. If you are bitten by an animal, you have to get one dose immediately and then additional doses on the third, seventh, fourteenth, and twenty-eighth day after that. Even if you've been previously vaccinated, you should get two more shots after you are bitten, one immediately and one three days later. Veterinarians and animal handlers should receive this series prophylactically.

Rotavirus. The vaccine prevents a gastrointestinal disease that is responsible for 55,000 to 70,000 hospitalizations and 20 to 60 deaths each year. Kids should get three doses at ages two, four, and six months. It hasn't been studied in kids older than six months, however.

Rubella (German measles). See above, under *Measles.*

Shingles. You can get herpes zoster, or shingles, if you have had either chicken pox or the chicken pox vaccine—it's caused by the same, dormant virus. The vaccine, approved in 2006, prevents about half of shingles cases, and can also reduce the pain caused by the blistering rash if you get the disease despite having been vaccinated. People over sixty should get a single dose.

Smallpox. The first vaccine invented. Vaccinations for smallpox have not been routinely given in the United States since 1980, when it was announced that the virus had been eradicated. The CDC issues complex procedures about vaccination in case of an epidemic. Not normally required except for laboratory workers who handle the virus.

Tetanus. See above, under *Diphtheria.*

Typhoid. Typhoid fever is caused by a bacterium in the genus Salmonella and is primarily spread through contaminated food or water. The vaccine isn't usually recommended within the United States, except for travelers to endemic areas and

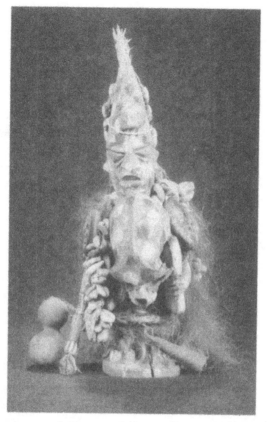

*A statue of Shapona, the West African god of
smallpox, carved by a traditional healer in 1969,
ten years before the disease was eradicated.*

for lab workers or others in close contact with a typhoid
carrier.

Varicella (chicken pox). Since 1995, the chicken pox vaccine
has helped reduce the number of school outbreaks of this virulent blistering virus. Kids should get two doses starting at
age one. Anyone older who has never had chicken pox should

get the shot, too. People who are immunocompromised should not get it, and pregnant women should wait until after they give birth.

Yellow fever. One of the oldest vaccines, it prevents a hemorrhagic viral fever with distinct jaundice symptoms. Only for people traveling to places, such as sub-Saharan Africa and South America, where yellow fever is endemic.

THE PERFECT CURE

God heals, and the doctor takes the fee.

—BENJAMIN FRANKLIN (1706–1790)

Take Two and Call in the Morning

ACETYLSALICYLIC ACID WAS INTRODUCED IN 1899 UNDER the trademark name Aspirin and is today probably the most widely used drug in the world. It is prescribed to treat the symptoms of rheumatoid arthritis, osteoarthritis, systemic lupus erythematosus, and other autoimmune diseases. People take it in its over-the-counter form to relieve pain from headaches, menstrual periods, arthritis, colds, toothaches, and muscle aches. It is used to prevent death in people who have had a heart attack or have the chest pain caused by angina, the failure of the heart to get enough oxygen. It prevents repeated strokes in people who have had one in the past. It is a very effective fever reducer. Americans consume about 29 billion aspirins every year. That's about ninety tablets a year for every man, woman, and child in the country—although children shouldn't take it because it is associated with Reye's syndrome, a rare and deadly disease of unknown cause and cure.

Prescription aspirin is available in an extended-release tablet, and it's available over the counter in pills, chewable tablets, chewing gum, and suppositories. You can also find it in combination with cold medicines, cough medicines, other pain relievers, and antacids.

Many people take small amounts of it daily—about 80 milligrams—because this has been shown to reduce the risk of heart attack and stroke. It's also used to treat rheumatic fever and Kawasaki disease, an illness of unknown cause that affects many organs and is particularly common in children.

Like any medicine, aspirin has side effects, most of them minor. It can cause nausea, vomiting, stomach pain, or a rash. But benign as it usually is, it can also cause some quite serious problems. Swelling of the lips and mouth, hives, difficulty breathing or talking, a fast heartbeat, cold skin, bloody vomit, blood in stool, ringing in the ears, and loss of hearing are all possible just from taking aspirin.

A problem with aspirin—and at the same time one of its virtues—is that it thins the blood. This helps prevent blood clots that lead to stroke and other problems, but it also increases the risk of internal bleeding. That's what causes the bloody vomit and stool, and if you bleed too much, you die.

The active ingredient in aspirin was first found in the bark of the willow tree, which contains high concentrations of salicin, a compound closely related to salicylic acid. Hippocrates was prescribing willow bark and leaves to treat pain and fever around 400 BC.

What might be considered the earliest scientific paper on

aspirin was published in 1763 by the Royal Society of London, a study by the Reverend Edward Stone called "Account of the Success of the Bark of the Willow in the Cure of Agues." (The paper's byline is "Edmund," but he signed himself "Edward.") Stone recounts his collection one summer of willow bark, "near a pound weight of it, which I dryed in a bag, upon the outside of a baker's oven, for more than three months, at which time it was to be reduced to a powder, by pounding and sifting after the manner that other barks are pulverized."

The reverend goes on to describe how he used the remedy for "agues and intermitting disorders," testing it on "fifty persons, and never failed in the cure, except in a few autumnal and quartan agues, with which the patients had been long and severely afflicted." He was very scientific in his procedures, administering the powder, "with any common vehicle, as water, tea, small beer and such like. This was done purely to ascertain its effects and that I might be assured the changes wrought in the patient could not be attributed to any other thing."

In the nineteenth century, scientists figured out how to synthesize the compound. The German drug company Friedrich Bayer & Co. perfected the technique, trademarked the name Aspirin, and began selling the medicine. Bayer still holds a trademark on the name in many countries, but not in the United States, where anyone can manufacture the substance and call it aspirin with a small *a*.

All brands of aspirin contain the same active ingredient: acetylsalicylic acid. No matter what you pay for aspirin, it's the same stuff, and despite repeated advertising claims to the contrary, no study has ever found that one brand is better or more effective than any another.

Reduce Your Risk by Drinking Coffee . . .

There are actually published studies, in respected medical journals, that show an association between drinking coffee and reducing the risk of disease. And it's not the caffeine but other ingredients in coffee that seem to be the reason.

Diabetes. Numerous studies demonstrate that drinking coffee reduces the risk of Type 2 diabetes, the kind usually contracted in adulthood. The authors are unsure why, but it probably has to do with the antioxidant content of coffee that helps control cell damage and with the chlorogenic acid that has been shown in animal studies to reduce glucose concentrations. Large quantities seem to be particularly effective—one study showed that more than six cups a day resulted in a decreased risk of 35 percent compared to those who drank two or fewer. There was no effect for drinking tea or other beverages with caffeine, so it is evidently some other ingredient in coffee that causes the effect.

Hypertension. Six cups or more of coffee a day may be helpful in reducing the risk for high blood pressure. One study showed that coffee abstainers had lower blood pressure than those who drank up to three cups a day, but higher than those who drank more than six cups.

Cirrhosis of the liver. There is apparently some ingredient in coffee—again, not necessarily caffeine—that offers protection against alcoholic cirrhosis of the liver. According to one study, there's also a reduced risk for liver cancer—one of the things that can follow from cirrhosis—in people who drink just one or two cups a day.

Heart disease. Here, the coffee effect is controversial. Generally, moderate coffee consumption is believed to decrease the risk of heart disease, but drinking large amounts may actually increase it. For the beneficial effect, researchers suspect that it's the antioxidants in coffee that are good for you.

. . . or Drinking Alcohol

Although the risks of too much drinking are well known, there are also many studies that show that drinking moderate amounts of alcohol can be a healthful activity, reducing the risk for the following:

Renal cancer. A review that pooled data from twelve studies covering more than 750,000 patients concluded that consuming one drink a day—of beer, liquor, or wine—would reduce the risk of renal cell carcinoma by about 28 percent compared to the risk among teetotalers.

Heart attack. A 2007 study demonstrates that men who drank one or two drinks a day—fifteen to thirty grams of alcohol— were 30 percent less likely to have a heart attack compared with those who drank none, and the more they drank, the more they appeared to reduce their risk—up to 60 percent for those who drank fifty grams a day, or a little more than three drinks. Another study suggested that women who had a drink a day reduced their risk of nonfatal heart attack, but that women who got drunk at least once a month were more than three times as likely to suffer a heart attack as abstainers. None of the authors, we should note, recommend that you take up drinking to prevent a heart attack.

Heart failure. In people age sixty-five and older, those who had a drink or two a day were about 16 percent less likely to suffer from heart failure or die from cardiac disease. The researchers followed these people for seven to ten years to record their alcohol consumption and health.

The Cranberry Juice Cure

The common belief is that cranberry juice prevents or cures urinary tract infections. This piece of folklore has a tiny grain of truth, just enough that some want to turn cranberry juice into a panacea.

The stuff has been studied scientifically—that is, in experiments in which one group of people susceptible to urinary infections drank cranberry juice and another group, similar in age, sex, health, and many other characteristics, took a placebo or another kind of juice or plain water. Then the researchers tracked their subjects—about one thousand people in ten different studies—to see who got urinary tract infections and who didn't.

The experiments showed that cranberry juice (or, in some of the studies, cranberry and lingonberry juice combined or cranberry tablets) reduced the incidence of urinary tract infections in some people by about 35 percent over a twelve-month period, compared with a placebo. People didn't like the cranberry preparations that much, and some had side effects like acid reflux, mild nausea, and frequent bowel movements. (Of course, as in all studies, people who took only the placebo complained that they had side effects, too—mostly headaches and nausea. Go figure.) Anyway, a lot of people dropped out of the studies, either because of side effects or for other reasons—moving away, having to go on other antibiotics, pregnancy, and so on.

But what about the people for whom the cranberries actually did some good? Well, for reasons that are unclear, women with recurrent infections seemed to get the most benefit, and the benefit they got was a reduction in the number of recurrent infections. It wasn't effective in elderly men and women, and it didn't work for people who had had urinary catheters inserted. Only one study suggested that the juice had any curative effect.

There were some problems with the studies. None of them had any justification for the dosages they administered, some of them didn't even describe the dosages in any clear and scientific way, and none made clear how long you have to keep drinking the juice or taking the cranberry tablets to get the benefit. In some of the studies, more than half of the participants dropped out, which makes you think that cranberry juice, whatever its theoretical advantages, isn't a very practical treatment in the real world. Children generally detested the stuff, citing the taste as the main reason for wanting to quit taking it.

There haven't been any studies at all that have compared cranberry juice with conventional antibiotic treatment for urinary tract infections, but apparently cranberries contain a substance that prevents bacteria from sticking to the walls of the bladder, which may help prevent infection. If it did work, cranberry juice could be preferable to antibiotics since it would be unlikely to create resistant strains of bacteria the way antibiotics almost inevitably do.

So there are still a lot of ifs here. If you're a woman with recurrent infections, if you don't have other health problems that would require antibiotics anyway, if you could figure out the right dosage and the right amount of time to keep on the regimen, if you don't get unpleasant side effects, and if you like the taste enough to stick with it, then cranberry juice could be a useful treatment. Even if the cranberry juice doesn't cure or prevent urinary infections, it's very unlikely to hurt you.

Why Chocolate Is Good for You

Happily, there is quite a bit of scientific evidence that chocolate is good for you, provided you don't overdo it, and provided you stick to dark chocolate.

In September 2008, a group of Italian researchers pointed out that the cocoa bean, from which chocolate is derived, is an extremely concentrated source of polyphenols, a type of antioxidant, and that evidence has been accumulating over the past decade that moderate consumption of dark chocolate may have protective effects against cardiovascular disease. They mentioned several mechanisms that might explain the effect. Polyphenols might have anti-inflammatory properties, might help prevent blood clots, might affect insulin sensitivity, might improve the function of the endothelial cells that line the blood vessels, and might lower blood pressure.

Other researchers summed up some of the evidence that chocolate might prevent hypertension in a review of five studies of the effect of dark chocolate on blood pressure. They concluded that in randomized, controlled trials in adults, diets rich in cocoa were associated with significant reductions in diastolic (the bottom number) and systolic (the top number) blood pressure. In fact, they found that it was in the same range as beta-blockers, the most common medicine given in cases of hypertension. They also found that there was a significant reduction in all-cause mortality for dark-chocolate eaters, suggesting that the stuff also confers some protection from heart disease.

Of course, the authors of the study warned people that this doesn't mean that it's a good idea to consume more chocolate than you're already consuming just because you think it might be good for your health. When we asked Dr. Dirk Taubert, the review's lead author, what he was doing himself, he confessed that he was eating more dark chocolate and he said that it made his blood pressure go down. "But," he said, "I have no dietary recommendations for others."

You don't like dark chocolate, only milk chocolate? You're out of luck. Milk proteins prevent the absorption of polyphenols, so milk chocolate doesn't have the same effect. It just tastes good.

Why Garlic Is Good for You

The beneficial effects of garlic have been known for centuries. Studies have shown that it reduces the risk for cardiovascular disease, reduces high blood pressure, controls cholesterol, and helps with blood coagulation. But why it does all these things has been something of a mystery.

Now researchers have figured out that garlic causes human red blood cells to produce hydrogen sulfide, a cardiovascular signaling molecule. Hydrogen sulfide is the same compound that makes rotten eggs smell awful, and in large quantities it's poisonous. But the effect in blood is beneficial— it helps relax the blood vessels and improve blood flow. This action accounts for the reduction in cardiovascular disease risk in people who eat it.

There aren't any other edible plants that contain the compounds—called allyl-substituted sulfur compounds—that produce this effect, so garlic is the only option.

B.O.

Yes, there's a long tradition of having a laugh about stinky people. It's certainly true that people can stink because they don't bathe properly. But sweat itself is odorless.

Here's what happens. There are two kinds of sweat glands, called eccrine and apocrine, that cover most of the body. Eccrine glands occur everywhere; apocrine glands are mostly in areas that grow lots of hair, like your armpits. If your body temperature rises—because of exercise or emotional arousal or any other reason—your nervous system tells your sweat glands to get into action. Sweat is mainly water, salt, and a few other electrolytes, and the evaporating moisture helps cool you down. When the sweat emerges on your skin, bacteria begin to break it down. As the bacteria eat up your sweat, they grow and excrete waste products. This stinks, especially the breakdown of the fatty sweat that comes out of the apocrine glands, which is one reason why armpits are particularly smelly.

All of that is normal. Take a bath, put on some deodorant, and the problem is solved. But there are also conditions, diseases, and disorders that cause body odors. First, there are people who, for genetic reasons, just sweat a lot. Inevitably, these people are going to have more problems with b.o. Any food that makes you sweat—hot drinks, hot soup, spicy food, alcohol, caffeine—will increase your chances of stinking. And eating some odoriferous spices may also produce body odors even without the additional problems caused by sweat—garlic and the Korean fermented vegetables called kimchi are notorious for this. There are drugs that cause sweating. Antipsychotic medicines, morphine, thyroid hormones, even aspirin and acetaminophen can do it.

Women going through menopause may sweat more when they have hot flashes, and men can have them, too, when they have reduced testosterone. Low blood sugar can make you sweat, and so can fevers. Leukemia, lymphoma, and tuberculosis can cause abnormal sweating and subsequent abnormal stinking.

Bad Morning Mouth

The origin of bad breath is almost always in the mouth, but there are also non-mouth problems that cause it, and we'll get to those in a minute. People with dental disease, especially infections of the gums called periodontal disease, can have bad breath, and it's the bacteria that are the cause. Leftover bits of food in your mouth can break down and cause odors. Certain foods like garlic and onions have volatile chemicals that stink. These can be smelled from bits in your mouth, but the chemicals also enter the bloodstream and are expelled through the lungs, so this is one kind of bad breath that doesn't start in your mouth—it only passes through on its way to the outside.

The "morning mouth" phenomenon is caused by dead cells that accumulate in your mouth while you're asleep and not producing enough saliva to clean things up. If you sleep with your mouth open, it gets even drier, and can cause more odors.

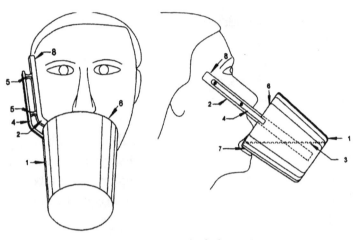

Hiccups: a new shock therapy?

Bad breath may be the least of the problems you'll encounter if you smoke.

Chronic infections of the lung can cause halitosis, as can some cancers. Kidney failure and liver failure produce characteristic bad breath odors. Chronic acid reflux can cause bad breath, as can sinus and throat infections.

A Cure for Hiccups

Apparently, a brown paper bag is no longer enough. On June 13, 2006, the U.S. Patent Office issued patent number 7062320 for this "apparatus for the treatment of hiccups involving galvanic stimulation of the Superficial Phrenetic and Vagus nerves using an electric current."

We think it sounds slightly more enjoyable than the "physiological cold block" method patented back in 1999.

CHAPTER

8

PREVENTION IS THE BEST MEDICINE

> The best doctors in the world are Doc-
> tor Diet, Doctor Quiet, and Doctor
> Merryman.
>
> —JONATHAN SWIFT (1667–1745)

The Healthiest Place to Live

DECIDING WHICH GEOGRAPHIC AREA IS "THE HEALTHIEST" involves plenty of subjective judgments. Is it healthier to live where there's a high crime rate if that place also has the best hospitals? Does a high concentration of doctors make a place healthier? Are you more likely to have an accident in some states than others? If a place has a high infant mortality rate but a low cancer rate, is it healthy to live there or not?

The United Health Foundation is a not-for-profit organization established by the large health care company United-Health Group, whose mission is to "improve the quality and cost effectiveness of medical outcomes, to expand access to health care services for those in challenging circumstances, and to enhance the well-being of communities." (A cynic might add that some other purposes are to improve the image of health insurance companies and make a lot of money, but let's not be cynical.)

The organization rates the U.S. states for health based on twenty different measures. These include "determinants" like smoking rates, obesity rates, number of children living in poverty, percent without health insurance, number of primary care physicians, and nine other such categories. They also include "health outcomes"—infant mortality, cardiovascular deaths, cancer deaths, premature death, and others. By adding up all these determinants and outcomes, they come up with a ranking for each state, and a percentage that each is above or below the national norm. The "score" indicates the percentage above or below the national average.

New England states all rank near the top. Mississippi ranks last. This does not mean that if you live in Mississippi, you will get healthy by moving to Vermont. On the other hand, it probably wouldn't hurt.

2007

Rank	State	Score
1	Vermont	21.7
2	Minnesota	20.5
3	Hawaii	19.5
4	New Hampshire	18.1
5	Connecticut	16.6
6	Utah	14.8
7	Maine	14.6
8	North Dakota	14.1
9	Massachusetts	13.5

Rank	State	Score
10	Nebraska	12.8
11	Rhode Island	12.5
12	Washington	12.2
12	Wisconsin	12.2
14	Iowa	10.7
15	Idaho	10.3
16	Colorado	9.7
16	South Dakota	9.7
18	Montana	9.5
19	Wyoming	8.6
20	Oregon	8.4
21	New Jersey	8.0
22	Virginia	6.3
23	Kansas	4.1
24	Pennsylvania	3.8
25	California	3.6
26	New York	3.1
27	Illinois	2.5
28	Maryland	1.8
29	Ohio	1.0
30	Alaska	0.1
31	Michigan	−0.6
32	Indiana	−0.7
33	Arizona	−1.7
34	Delaware	−2.8
35	Missouri	−3.4
36	North Carolina	−4.7
37	Texas	−5.5
38	New Mexico	−5.9
39	Nevada	−7.3

Rank	State	Score
40	Georgia	−8.5
41	Florida	−8.8
42	South Carolina	−10.1
43	Kentucky	−10.6
44	West Virginia	−11.8
45	Alabama	−11.9
46	Tennessee	−14.0
47	Oklahoma	−14.7
48	Arkansas	−16.3
49	Louisiana	−18.6
50	Mississippi	−19.6

Poisoned

If you want to avoid dying from poisoning, you should also let geography be your guide. Why people in the Southwest keep poisoning themselves and others, we don't know, but the upper Midwest looks like a good place to avoid swallowing something deadly. Poisoning is the second leading cause of accidental death in the United States, exceeded only by traffic accidents. For some reason, West Virginia has the highest rate of poisoning death of all the states—19.4 per 100,000, followed closely by New Mexico, Utah, and Nevada. In 2004, 90 percent of poisonings were caused by drugs, 7 percent by inhalation of gases and vapors, 1 percent by alcohol, and 1 percent by all other substances. Homicide by poison accounted for 0.3 percent of deaths.

Death by Poisoning

Per 100,000 population, 2004

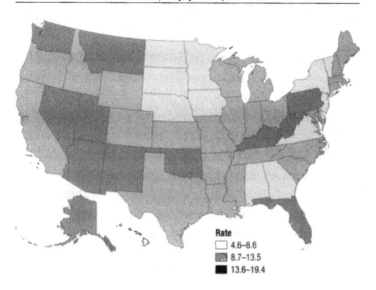

Rate
- ☐ 4.6–8.6
- ▨ 8.7–13.5
- ■ 13.6–19.4

Thank You for Not Smoking

It took more than nine hundred pages for the latest edition of the *Surgeon General's Report on the Health Consequences of Smoking* to describe all the harm smoking can do and what might be done to reduce it. Here are twenty-five diseases the report says are proven to be linked to smoking:

Lung cancer	Bladder cancer
Laryngeal cancer	Kidney cancer
Mouth cancer	Ovarian cancer
Pharyngeal cancer	Cervical cancer
Esophageal cancer	Endometrial cancer
Pancreatic cancer	Stomach cancer

Colorectal cancer	Coronary heart disease
Prostate cancer	Cerebrovascular disease
Acute leukemia	Abdominal aortic aneurysm
Liver cancer	Acute respiratory illness
Brain cancer	Chronic respiratory disease
Breast cancer	Peptic ulcer disease
Atherosclerosis	

Tobacco smoke contains more than a hundred known carcinogens. Nicotine gets into your brain within ten seconds after you inhale smoke, and, along with lots of other poisons in tobacco, is distributed throughout the body; it has been found in breast milk and cervical mucus. Carbon monoxide moves from the lungs to the capillaries, where it binds to the oxygen-transporting hemoglobin in red blood cells. Benzopyrene, another carcinogen in tobacco smoke, can be found in the blood cells, airway cells, and the major organs of smokers. Smoking increases the risk for infections of the respiratory tract and other organs. Because it causes oxidative stress, which is probably one mechanism that underlies aging and many chronic diseases associated with aging, it also, in a sense, makes you older.

Smoking during pregnancy causes birth defects, infant mortality, and child physical and mental developmental problems. Smoking leads to dental problems like periodontitis and dental cavities. It reduces bone density, leading to fractures.

Smokers don't sleep well. They spend less time in deep sleep and more time in light sleep than nonsmokers, and the greatest differences are in the early stages of sleep. Scientists suggest that smokers are undergoing nicotine withdrawal every night, which causes their problems.

There's more. It causes cataracts, age-related macular degeneration (which can lead to blindness), and an increased risk for diabetic retinopathy, which can also make you blind. It causes glaucoma, too. Oh, yeah—it also interferes with circulation, which can cause erectile dysfunction. And it makes your skin prematurely wrinkled.

Secondhand Smoke

Here's the really great thing about tobacco: you don't even have to smoke the stuff for it to make you sick. All you have to do is habitually sit (or stand or lie) near someone who does. In 2006, the Surgeon General issued a report on secondhand smoke, which concluded that there is no safe level of exposure and that exposure causes many of the same disorders and diseases that smoking causes. It's particularly harmful to children, in whom it can cause lower respiratory illnesses, middle ear infections, asthma, and lung growth problems, not to mention fetal growth impairment, spontaneous abortions, preterm delivery, low birth weight, and sudden infant death syndrome. And it's a good way to kill your wife or husband, too: spouses of smokers have an increased risk of stroke.

Looking for some good news about secondhand smoke? Although smoking certainly increases the risk for infertility, the evidence that secondhand smoke does so is weak, and the evidence linking it to childhood cancers is only suggestive. When it comes to smoking, that is about as good as it gets.

Can You Prevent Your Skin from Wrinkling?

Nostrums to prevent skin from wrinkling are among the best-selling products of snake-oil salesmen everywhere, but oddly enough, there are three that are actually known to make skin less wrinkled. These treatments aren't available over the counter, however, and you will probably have to visit a dermatologist to get the benefits. None of them lasts forever, but there's good scientific evidence for them, and if the problem really bothers you, you might want to try them.

Skin wrinkles because the dermal collagen—the stuff that gives skin its structure—gets fragmented with sun exposure and age. The fibroblasts, which produce collagen, begin to fail, producing less collagen and more enzymes that degrade collagen. So the key to any treatment is stimulating the production of new, nonfragmented and undamaged collagen and reducing the production of the collagen-destroying enzyme.

Here are proven treatments for preventing or repairing wrinkled skin:

Topical application of retinoic acid. Retinoic acid, a form of vitamin A, was the first topical treatment shown to improve the appearance of wrinkled skin. Although no one is quite sure how it does it, retinoic acid—and some of its chemical cousins, retinol and retinal—cause the deposition of new, undamaged collagen in both aging and sun-damaged skin. There are various products on the market that contain retinol, but most of the stuff you can buy over the counter doesn't work because the concentrations aren't high enough. Generally speaking, you're going to need a prescription for a cream containing 0.2 to 0.6 percent retinol. Unfortunately, the medicine at this concentration can have side effects, including a nasty rash. If a rash occurs, you have to stop using the cream. The other drawback is that retinol makes the skin more sensitive to light, so you have to be very careful about sun exposure when you're using it.

Carbon dioxide laser resurfacing. A doctor can use a laser to remove a thin layer of skin without damaging the nearby tissue. Essentially this causes a wound that has to heal. As it heals, which can take two to three weeks, new collagen is laid down. It works because it causes high levels of an enzyme that destroys fragmented collagen. Then it reduces the levels of this enzyme, which encourages the production of new collagen. It's a techique that can also be used to remove warts and birthmarks. The wounded skin requires some care to prevent scarring. As it heals, you have to clean it often with saline or a dilute solution of vinegar. If you do it right, the effect lasts for many years.

Hyaluronic acid injections. Researchers found this one accidentally. Originally, it was used as a space filler, just to plump up places that needed extra material—it wasn't supposed to have any physiological effect. But then dermatologists noticed that as the injected material stretches the skin, the skin reacts by producing more collagen and less of the enzyme that destroys it. About a month after the injection, you begin to see the effects. But after six months, the effect fades, and you have to do it again. There are some skin creams that have hyaluronic acid in them, but it's not the same type. Rubbing hyaluronic acid on your skin has no known effect.

What a First Aid Kit Is Supposed to Have in It

The American College of Emergency Physicians wants you to be prepared. First, it wants you take a first aid class and a class in cardiopulmonary resuscitation (CPR). Then it wants you to keep certain things in a first aid kit. Everything on this list is available at a pharmacy without a prescription. A cloth tote bag is recommend to put it all in. You're supposed to keep the kit where kids can't reach it and check it regularly to make sure everything is there and none of the medicines are out of date.

Information. In the kit, you should have the emergency phone numbers for your family physician and pediatrician, the regional Poison Control Center, and, if 911 doesn't function where you are, the numbers of the police, fire department, and ambulance service. The kit should include complete medical consent forms for your family, to allow someone to authorize medical treatment in an emergency when you're unable to give consent.

You also should keep a list of the contents of the kit, a list of allergies each member of the family has, and a list of medications used by each member of the family.

Medicines and supplies. Acetaminophen (Tylenol or a generic equivalent), ibuprofen (Advil, Motrin, or a generic equivalent), and aspirin. The aspirin is not just for headaches but should be given in case of a heart attack. Also:

Cough suppressant
Antihistamine
Decongestant tablets
Oral medicine syringe (to administer oral medicine to children)
Fluids for oral rehydration when treating infant diarrhea
Assorted-size bandages
Bandage closures (butterfly bandages) for taping edges of cuts together

A triangular bandage for making a sling
Elastic wraps for wrist, ankle, and elbow injuries
Gauze in two- and four-inch rolls
Gauze pads
Adhesive tape
Scissors
Safety pins
Antiseptic wipes
Disposable cold packs
Tweezers
Hydrogen peroxide for disinfecting wounds
Gloves for protecting hands and reducing risk of infection
    when treating wounds
Thermometer
Petroleum jelly for lubricating a rectal thermometer
Calamine lotion
Hydrocortisone cream for relieving irritation from rashes

And if someone in the family has a life-threatening allergy, you should carry appropriate medicine for it.

Who Gets Bitten by Venomous Snakes?

There are poisonous snakes on every continent except Antarctica, six hundred different species that immobilize their prey with venom, a modified form of saliva, injected through hollow fangs. They also use the poisonous fangs in self-defense, which is how humans usually get bitten—snakes don't generally regard humans as prey.

Snakebites are not a small problem. One study estimated that worldwide there are 421,000 snakebites and 20,000 deaths

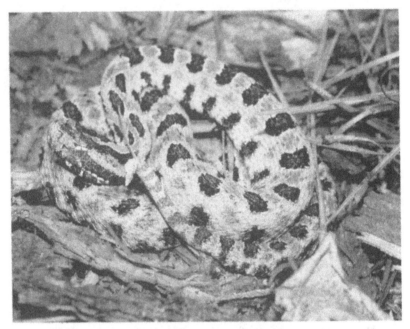

A Carolina pygmy rattlesnake. W. C. Fields once said, "Always carry a flagon of whiskey in case of snakebite and furthermore always carry a small snake."

from them every year. Most of the bites occur in South and Southeast Asia and in sub-Saharan Africa. India alone accounts for more than half of the snakebite deaths.

Americans are not immune. About 8,000 people in the United States are bitten by poisonous snakes each year, and somewhere between fourteen and twenty people die from the bites. More than 80 percent of the bites in California in 2002 were from a species called *Crotalus viridis helleri*, the Southern Pacific rattlesnake. Most victims of snakebite are male, between the ages of seventeen and twenty-seven. About 28 percent of the victims were drunk, or at least had been consuming alcohol at the time of the incident. Ninety-eight percent of bites occur on the hands or arms, and they are almost never the result of an unprovoked snake attack—most resulted from deliberate attempts to handle, harm, or kill a snake.

In a group of snakebite victims studied by researchers, 40 percent treated the wound, or had it treated by someone else, by tying on a tourniquet; 35 percent made a cut in the wound, generally using whatever sharp instrument was available; and 44 percent sucked on the wound, usually using their mouths. Tying a tourniquet doesn't do any good, and if it is tied too tightly, it can affect blood supply and cause considerable harm to the affected limb. Incision and suction do not weaken the power of the venom, and because incisions are usually made by panicked people with no surgical expertise and using nonsterile equipment, they often result in secondary infections. The best first aid for snakebite is to move the victim at a safe speed to a hospital that is equipped with a supply of antivenin and a knowledgeable staff.

So the fact is that most people who are afraid of getting bitten by a snake have little to fear. If you don't get drunk and start messing with a rattlesnake, you'll probably be fine.

Total Snakebite Deaths in the United States

Year	Deaths
1999	7
2000	12
2001	7
2002	3
2003	2
2004	6

Unhealthy Behavior

"Physically inactive" means never engaging in any exercise; "obese" means a body mass index above 30. The sleep numbers are for a twenty-four-hour day.

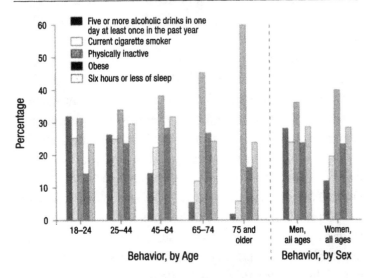

Behavior, by Age | Behavior, by Sex

Unhealthful Behavior

Who is most at risk for unhealthful behavior? First, you need to know what counts as unhealthful. Physical inactivity—never engaging in any exercise—is one. So is having a body mass index (an estimate of body fat based on your height and weight) of greater than thirty. And so does how much sleep you get in a twenty-four-hour period. (For more on the connection between sleep and health, see chapter 11.)

Who Doesn't Get Enough Exercise?

Get that "who me?" look off your face, because we know who you are. And now we're going to tell on you. The

CDC runs a continuing survey to see who's been naughty, and it tracks lots of bad behavior—smoking, binge drinking, failure to use seat belts, being overweight, and so on. One of the bad behaviors it's interested in is being a couch potato.

The CDC doesn't demand that you participate in a triathlon or do a hundred one-handed push-ups, either. All it asks is whether you spent any leisure time at all in physical activity—for example, running, doing calisthenics, golfing, gardening, or walking—in the last month. The number of Americans not even doing that much, it turns out, is large.

The likelihood that you're one of them varies depending on what state you live in. Nationally, more than 22 percent of Americans get virtually no exercise. For some reason, people in Minnesota are more active than in any other state—only 14.2 percent were lazing around when the CDC came calling. At the other extreme was Louisiana, with 31 percent of residents having done nothing in the previous month that threatened to increase their pulse above the resting level.

The CDC recommends that people engage in thirty minutes of moderate physical activity on most days and preferably every day, and they did a survey to find out if people were listening to this advice. Most of them weren't.

True, when they compared numbers for 2001 with those for 2005, they found that people were exercising slightly more—the prevalence of regular exercise among women increased 8.6 percent and among men 3.5 percent. But still only a minority of people were getting enough exercise.

It also found that how much exercise you get depends on ethnicity and education level: people without a high school diploma exercise the least, and those who've graduated from college exercise the most. White people exercise more than

Hispanic people, and Hispanic people more than black people. Men exercise more than women.

Percentage of Adults Who Reported Meeting the
***Healthy People 2010* Objective for Physical Activity, 2005**

Objective: At least thirty minutes of moderate-intensity activity on five or more days a week, or at least twenty minutes a day of vigorous-intensity activity on three or more days a week, or both.

	Men	Women
Age group (years)		
18–24	62.0	52.7
25–34	51.5	50.5
35–44	49.6	49.7
45–64	46.5	45.5
65 or older	44.5	36.3
Race/ethnicity		
White, non-Hispanic	52.3	49.6
Black, non-Hispanic	45.3	36.1
Hispanic	41.9	40.5
Other race	45.7	46.6
Education level		
Less than high school graduate	37.2	37.1
High school graduate	47.9	43.2
Some college	54.6	53.3
College graduate	54.6	53.3
Total	**49.7**	**46.7**

Source: Behavioral Risk Factor Surveillance System, United States, 2005

Watching Their Weight

Kids are getting fatter, boys even more so than girls.

Percentage of Overweight Kids, Ages Two to Nineteen

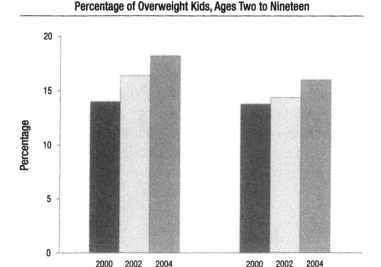

Jobs That Are Bad for Your Health

People who work for the U.S. Postal Service are always "going postal," shooting up the place, so being a mailman must be a pretty dangerous job, right? Actually, no. The CDC reports that postal workers are no more likely to be murdered than anyone else. You probably hear about (and pay attention to) more postal worker homicides mostly because there are more postal workers than most other kinds of employees, and the post office is a place we're all familiar with that most of us visit from time to time. The death rate among postal workers is in fact less than half the rate for all industries combined. There are postal workers who have been murdered on the job, of course, but the rate of homicide among them is lower than the average for all workers. Most of the people who die on the job as postal workers are killed in motor vehicle accidents.

Catching lobsters in Maine, on the other hand—now there's a good way to gamble with your life. From 1993 to 1997, the occupational fatality rate for lobstermen in Maine was 14 per 100,000, more than two and a half times the national average of 4.8 for all industries. Lobstermen tend to get tangled in the ropes that hold the lobster pots, get pulled overboard, and drown. The National Institute for Occupa-

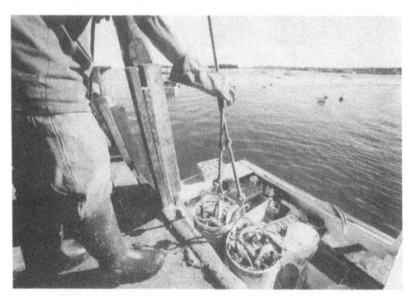

Lobstering: a really dangerous job, depending on how you do the math.

tional Safety and Health reports one grisly incident in which a lobsterman working alone was pulled into the water when the line wrapped around his wrist. They found him, dead, when another lobsterman saw his boat circling aimlessly. He had cut the line around his wrist, but then he was apparently unable to climb back into his moving boat.

Fishing may be among the most dangerous professions, with logging close by, but it is not easy to conclude from the numbers which occupations are the most dangerous, because "most dangerous" is an opinion, not a statistical category. For example, let's imagine some job that only one thousand people engage in—say, art restorers who work in museums (we're making this up as we go along). Suppose that one of them fell off a ladder and died. That would make the rate of death for that profession 100 per 100,000, but no one would believe that restoring art in museums is a job that falls between fishing and logging for risk of death. Rates per 100,000 can be deceptive, so you really have to look at the numbers in various ways to get a true picture.

The two charts on the next page give a general idea—but a general idea only—of how dangerous various jobs and various industries are.

Occupational Hazards

Number and rate of fatal injuries by industry, 2007

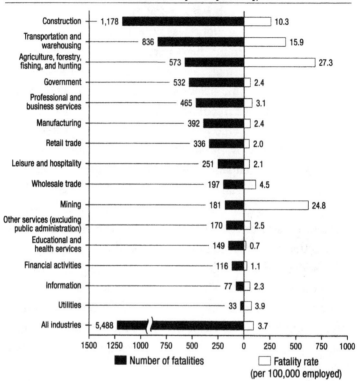

Industry	Number of fatalities	Fatality rate (per 100,000 employed)
Construction	1,178	10.3
Transportation and warehousing	836	15.9
Agriculture, forestry, fishing, and hunting	573	27.3
Government	532	2.4
Professional and business services	465	3.1
Manufacturing	392	2.4
Retail trade	336	2.0
Leisure and hospitality	251	2.1
Wholesale trade	197	4.5
Mining	181	24.8
Other services (excluding public administration)	170	2.5
Educational and health services	149	0.7
Financial activities	116	1.1
Information	77	2.3
Utilities	33	3.9
All industries	5,488	3.7

■ Number of fatalities □ Fatality rate (per 100,000 employed)

Some Jobs with High Fatality Rates

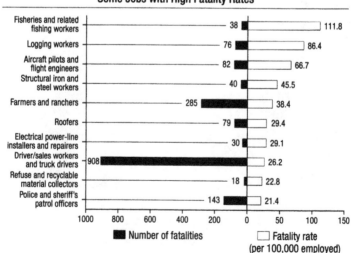

Job	Number of fatalities	Fatality rate (per 100,000 employed)
Fisheries and related fishing workers	38	111.8
Logging workers	76	86.4
Aircraft pilots and flight engineers	82	66.7
Structural iron and steel workers	40	45.5
Farmers and ranchers	285	38.4
Roofers	79	29.4
Electrical power-line installers and repairers	30	29.1
Driver/sales workers and truck drivers	908	26.2
Refuse and recyclable material collectors	18	22.8
Police and sheriff's patrol officers	143	21.4

■ Number of fatalities □ Fatality rate (per 100,000 employed)

9

INVENTION IS THE BEST MEDICINE

*First the doctor told me the good news:
I was going to have a disease named
after me.*

—STEVE MARTIN (B. 1945)

Medical Firsts

First surgery. What counts as surgery—and what counts as
first, for that matter—can be argued. But a jawbone found in
Egypt and dated about 2650 BC had two perforations below the
root of the first molar, suggesting that someone was trying to
drain an abscessed tooth. The oldest known surgery text was
written by the Indian physician Sushruta around 600 BC. It describes various kinds of surgery and includes instructions on
how to do a nose job, among other cosmetic procedures. Until
the twentieth century, when doctors figured out how to control
bleeding, infection, and pain effectively, even minor surgery
was a fairly dicey proposition.

First vaccine. Everyone knows that Edward Jenner (1749–1823) invented the smallpox vaccine in 1796, but actually a half dozen people had successfully used cowpox to vaccinate people against smallpox before Jenner's work. Jenner perfected the technique. It was almost a hundred years before anyone developed another vaccine, the one for cholera in 1879.

First stethoscope. The tool was invented in 1816 by a French doctor, René T. H. Laënnec (1781–1826). He was also trained as a flautist, which may help explain his interest in listening to the music inside the human body.

First syringe. There's nothing new about the principle of injection. Doctors have been injecting stuff into people for hundreds, maybe even thousands, of years. But until the mid-nineteenth century, they did it through natural openings of the body, or through a cut made in the skin. The hollow needle invented in 1844 by an Irish physician named Francis Rynd (1811–1861) was the first tool that looked like a modern syringe. A Frenchman, Charles-Gabriel Chavaz, developed a practical metal syringe about 1853. Of course, the germ theory of disease was yet to be widely accepted, and there is a high probability that using these first needles did more harm than good.

First cesarean section. Julius Caesar was almost certainly not born by cesarean section. According to scholars at the National Library of Medicine, babies in ancient Rome were from their mothers' wombs untimely ripp'd only when the mother was dead or dying, and Caesar's mother apparently lived at least until Caesar invaded Britain. Although Roman law in Caesar's time did decree that all women in danger of dying should

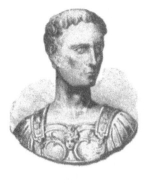

Caesar: a normal vaginal birth.

be cut open in order to save the baby, a different explanation for the term seems more plausible: the Latin word for "cut" is *caedere*, and babies born by postmortem operations were called *caesones*.

There are records of cesarean birth dating back to antiquity, although most details, such as which babies or mothers died and which ones lived, are, to say the least, somewhat unreliably reported. There are also accounts of cesarean sections carried out by indigenous peoples. The earliest cesareans took place without the help of doctors or hospitals—and a good thing, too, considering the sanitary conditions in hospitals prior to the early twentieth century. It's probably impossible to say when the first successful cesarean was performed— successful in the sense that both mother and child survived— but it was almost certainly a long, long time ago.

By 2007, about 31.8 percent of babies born in the United States were born by cesarean, the largest proportion of cesarean births reported to date. Since 1996, the cesarean rate has increased by 46 percent, both because there are more first births by cesarean and because there are fewer vaginal deliveries by women who have had a cesarean.

First artificial insemination. The first documented artificial insemination was performed by Lazzaro Spallanzani (1729– 1799), an Italian biologist who in 1784 inseminated a dog who gave birth to three puppies two months later. Over the next couple of centuries, all sorts of domestic animals were

Percentage of Births by Cesarean Delivery

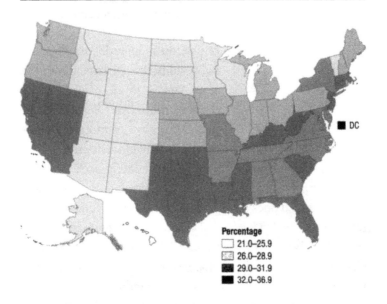

■ DC

Percentage
☐ 21.0–25.9
▨ 26.0–28.9
▨ 29.0–31.9
■ 32.0–36.9

artificially inseminated by hundreds of researchers, animal breeders, and farmers. But who cares? You wanted to know when the first *human* artificial insemination took place. That's a little harder to say, partly because it depends on what you mean by "artificial." Almost certainly, attempts were made to insert sperm into women in other than the usual way long before the twentieth century. There is a report in a 1953 issue of the French medical journal *Le progrès médical* describing a human artificial insemination, which may be the first documented report of the procedure. But until the late 1960s or early '70s, the procedure was at best uncommon. Most sources cite Louise Brown, born on July 25, 1978, as the first "test-tube baby"—that is, the product of an insemination that took place entirely outside the human body.

First blood transfusion. Although the story is disputed by some, in 1492 Stefano Infessura reported that Pope Innocent VIII received a blood transfusion from three ten-year-old boys. The pope died, and so did the boys. By the seventeenth century, there was quite a lot of blood being transfused between animals. Then in 1667, Jean-Baptiste Denys transfused some sheep blood into a human who, remarkably, survived.

Probably the first successful human transfusion was performed in 1818 by James Blundell (1791–1878), an obstetrician who transfused blood from a man into his wife. Half of Blundell's transfused patients died—but on the other hand, half of them survived. By the early twentieth century, techniques for storing blood at low temperatures and using anticoagulants to prevent it from clotting were being widely used. In 1909, Karl Landsteiner discovered the now well-known A, B, AB, and O groups and showed how problems develop (or don't develop) depending on what blood groups are being transfused to which individuals.

First prosthesis. The oldest known functional prosthesis is a bronze leg dating from about 300 BC that was found in Capua, Italy. The leg was held at the Royal College of Surgeons in London but was destroyed by Luftwaffe bombs during World War II.

But in 2007, British researchers announced that they were recruiting toeless volunteers to test a replica of what they suspected was an even older prosthetic, an artificial toe attached to a mummy dating from 1000 to 600 BC. The toe, which the researchers said showed signs of wear, was attached to the foot of a woman aged between fifty and sixty years.

A 2,400-year-old artificial leg.

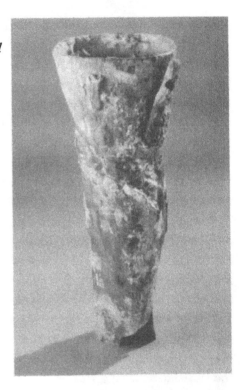

First dental implant. In a Mayan burial site in Honduras in 1931, archaeologists found the jawbone of a woman who had had three pieces of shell placed in her lower jaw, apparently to replace missing teeth. The bones date from about 600 AD. In 1970, a Brazilian dental academic, Amadeo Bobbio, studied the specimens and, noting bone growth around the shells, concluded that the implants were placed during life.

Modern dental implants are made of titanium, not seashells. In 1965, Per-Ingvar Brånemark (b. 1929), a professor of anatomy at Gothenburg University in Sweden, placed the first titanium dental implant into a human volunteer, a Swede named Gösta Larsson. The device is usually composed of a screw that is drilled into the bone and a crown that looks like a tooth. The screw is implanted and the site is allowed to heal and become integrated into the bone of the jaw before the crown is attached.

First successful organ transplant. On December 23, 1954, Joseph Murray and David Hume transplanted a kidney from one identical twin to another at Peter Bent Brigham Hospital in Boston. The twin with the new kidney lived another eight years, and Murray collected the Nobel Prize in 1990 for his efforts. Other organs followed: the first lung transplant in 1963, the first liver and heart transplants in 1967. In 1981, Norman Shumway at Stanford University did the first heart/lung transplant; in 1988 the first small intestine was transplanted. Surgeons have been trying to put animal organs into humans for more than a hundred years, but without success. In 1992 a baboon liver was transplanted into a thirty-five-year-old man. The man died of a stroke shortly afterward.

First artificial heart. Lively dispute here. Mechanical hearts and blood purifiers were first used in the 1950s, but William DeVries (b. 1943), an American surgeon, implanted the first artificial heart in a patient in 1982. This was the one perfected by Robert Jarvik, but he didn't actually invent it—he worked on and improved a device first invented and patented in 1963 by Paul Winchell (1922–2005)—the same Paul Winchell who was a TV comedian and ventriloquist in the 1950s and '60s. Winchell donated the patent, number 3097366, to the University of Utah. Dr. Jarvik explains this matter quite differently on his Web site, denying that Winchell's invention had anything to do with his.

Cut and Paste

New heart, new liver, new lungs, new pancreas, new intestines, new bones, tendons, corneas, heart valves, veins, arms, and skin, even a complete new face. If yours is broke, we can swap it out for a new one. Where do we get the spare parts? Usually from people who no longer need them—that is, they're dead. Sometimes a living person can help you out, but less often. Who can give and who can get varies by organ.

Kidneys, livers, intestines, lungs, bones, and certain parts of the pancreas can be donated by people who are still alive, but it's a lot easier if they're not. Blood transfusions have to come from living people, and so do bone marrow transplants, but those two are the only current transplant procedures that require that the donor be alive and actively consent to the procedure.

An organ has to be in good shape if it's going to be moved into a new person, and requirements vary depending on what organ you're replacing. A heart, for example, does best if it comes from a woman. The age of the heart doesn't seem to affect the survival of the person who receives it, except that older hearts are more likely to have various problems that might make them ineligible. The surgeons will examine the heart to make sure it's a good one, and may want to know something about the medical history of the donor to make sure he or she didn't have too many risk factors for heart disease. Heart transplants aren't undertaken lightly, but when they're done they work pretty well. About 85 percent of heart transplant patients are still alive one year, and 75 percent three years, after the operation.

Heart transplants occur about 2,000 times a year in the United States. There have even been a few living heart donors—this can be done if a person gives his heart to someone and gets a replacement from a cadaver. The first one of these in the United States was done in 1987, and there have been thirty-nine more since then. This happens when a person needs a lung transplant but has a healthy heart. He receives a heart-lung transplant from a cadaver (less risky than transplanting the lungs alone) and then donates his healthy heart to another person.

About 16,000 kidneys are transplanted every year. Of these, around 10,000 come from dead people, the rest from living donors. For almost 2,000 patients, the kidney is a repeat transplant. There isn't an official age limit for donating a kidney, and people who receive kidneys from people over sixty do just about as well as people who get them from younger donors.

There are around 6,500 liver transplants a year, and only about 250 are from living donors, most of them blood relations of the recipient who contribute a part of their livers. Again, there aren't any restrictions on the age of the donor—the main requirements are that the livers of the donor and recipient be about the same size and that people have compatible blood types. According to the American Liver Foundation, at any given time there are around 17,000 people waiting for a liver. The sickest patients move to the top of the list.

Pancreas transplants are uncommon—about 500 are done each year. There is an experimental procedure by which a living donor can give certain pancreatic cells to another person, but this has been done only twenty-three times since 1988. Donors older than forty-five are generally considered ineligible. About 850 times a year a combination kidney and pancreas transplant is done. When this is done, the organs are almost always taken from cadavers.

It is possible to transplant a lung from a living patient, but the operation is rarely done. It's tricky, because at least two people have to contribute parts of their lung to make an entire new lung for the recipient, but it's often successful because the donors are closely related and because the recipient can begin taking immunosuppressive medicine while the operation is being planned—it's not done on an emergency basis as is the case with a cadaver donor. About 1,400 lungs are transplanted from cadavers. Donors generally have to be under age fifty-five, and, of course, their lungs have to be healthy and free of bacteria, fungus, and a significant number of white blood cells (which would indicate infection). Until 1989, according to the American Lung Association, it was common to do a combined heart and lung transplant, but now single lung transplants are the most common form. There are about thirty heart-lung transplants a year in the United States.

An intestine that is lost in an accident or stops functioning because of disease can be replaced, but it's not a common operation. About 175 intestine transplants are done a year; 35 of them have been from living donors since 1995.

No one is automatically ruled out for donating corneas. As long as the donor and the cornea are generally healthy, it doesn't matter how old the person it came from was. It just has to be collected quickly after death. Corneas are the most commonly transplanted of all organs—about 40,000 of them are done every year.

Bone can be replaced as an autograft—that is, with bone from your own body—or as an allograft, meaning bone from another person's body. Bone marrow cell transplants are done to treat leukemia, multiple myeloma, aplastic anemia, and several other diseases, but the donor has to be carefully matched to the recipient, and this is often extremely difficult to do. There are around 8,000 transplants a year of bone marrow cells from one person to another. Cells can be taken from a person, treated outside the body, and then put back into the same person. This is done about 11,000 times a year.

Fixed Up

In addition to artificial arms, legs, fingers, and toes, a number of devices can be implanted inside the body to make things work better. Depending on the device, they can be powered by either internal batteries or an external power source. And some devices are powered only by the person in whom they are implanted.

Millions of people have metal of one kind or another implanted in their bodies. With more than 6 million people having had total hip or knee replacements between 1991 and 2004 (the most recent figures available at this writing from the American Academy of Orthopaedic Surgeons), plus all the pacemakers, defibrillators, and other kinds of machinery, this can make for a long wait at the security gate metal detector. In one study, 90 percent of people with orthopedic implants set off the alarms.

The Transportation Security Administration recommends that people with pacemakers tell the security guard they have one and carry a "Pacemaker Identification Card." But the guard will still pat you down. It is "recommended, but not required" that you tell the guard where your implant is. If you're worried that the X-ray machine will affect your device, you can ask for a pat-down instead. If you don't want the assembled multitudes to know about your implant, the

TSA says, you can "ask the Security Officer to please be discreet when assisting you through the screening process." They don't say what happens if you don't say please. In any case, if the security people can't figure out why you're setting off the alarm, you won't get on the plane.

You might want to get to the airport early, whether you have an implanted medical device or not.

Cardiac pacemakers for conduction disorders of the heart (brachycardia). The first pacemakers, in the 1950s, had a lead that ran from the heart to the machine, which was outside the body, and the machine had to be plugged into the wall. This considerably limited the mobility of patients who needed them. The first battery-powered pacemaker appeared in 1957, and by 1960 the totally implantable device had been developed. It had a battery that had to be replaced every year and a half or so. By the mid-1960s, surgeons had developed techniques to insert the devices without having to open the chest cavity. The leads were inserted through a vein leading to the heart and the device itself could be implanted under the skin. A few years later, "demand" pacemakers were developed, devices that provided an assist only when needed.

By the 1970s, there were pacemakers with extended-life batteries that could last as long as ten years, titanium casings that shielded the devices from external electromagnetic interference, and pacemakers that could work on more than one chamber of the heart at the same time. Today, pacemakers can be programmed remotely, automatically adjust for physical activity, recognize and adjust for abnormal activity in the heart, and collect information and store it for future reference. And they are half the size of earlier devices.

Cardiac defibrillators for ventricular and atrial tachyarrhythmia and fibrillation. Different from pacemakers, these devices provide an electric shock to the heart to restore normal beats when the heart begins to beat irregularly—similar to the defibrillation paddles used by medical personnel and featured in almost every episode of most TV medical dramas.

The first implantable defibrillators appeared in the 1980s with batteries that lasted about a year. They provided a shock of a single magnitude. By the 1990s, refinements allowed the devices to produce variable shocks depending on the severity of the arrhythmia detected, and surgeons could put in the leads through a vein, as they had been doing for some time with pacemakers, eliminating the need for opening the chest cavity. Smaller devices were introduced that could be implanted in the upper chest, and microcomputers in the devices allowed storing of data so that doctors could monitor heart function. Now there are devices that can regulate heartbeats that are too slow as well as too fast.

Left ventricular assist devices. Used to help a failing left ventricle pump blood out of the heart, these are often used in people waiting for heart transplants. The device has a tube that pulls blood out of the left ventricle into a pump and then moves it into the aorta to start circulating blood around the body. The pump is implanted near the top of the abdomen with a tube extending through the abdominal wall to the battery and controls. People can live outside the hospital with the devices for several months with a reasonable degree of comfort. The first of these devices was approved by the FDA in October 1994. Improvements in the pumping mechanism and reductions in size have made the devices much more efficient than the earliest models. Researchers are now experimenting with eliminating the cables by using transcutaneous induction to power the pump.

Neurological stimulators. Brain stimulators treat essential tremor, a movement disorder in which the patient trembles uncontrollably while engaging in activities such as eating, drinking, or using a pen or pencil. The patient is awake during surgery to implant the electrodes, and his or her cooperation is essential in getting them in the right place. After the surgery the device is programmed, by trial and error, in cooperation with the patient, to produce the best results. The FDA approved the first deep brain stimulator in 1997 to treat both essential tremor and the tremor of Parkinson's disease.

Drug pumps. In use since the early 1980s, an infusion pump is placed under the skin in the abdominal area, and a catheter is inserted into the spine so that pain-relieving medicine can be pumped directly into the cerebrospinal fluid. With this method the medicine is effective at much smaller doses, since it doesn't have to circulate through the blood.

Heart valves. There are two kinds of heart valves: mechanical and biological. Mechanical valves, made of metal, plastics, and other synthetic materials, require that the patient take blood-thinning drugs for the rest of his or her life. Valve replacements in the United States are usually done using material taken from a horse or cow pericardial sac or harvested from human cadavers. The material is treated in such a way that the patient's immune system will not reject it, and blood-thinning drugs are not usually required. The valves are inserted during open-heart surgery.

Artificial joints. Now a common method of treating bone diseases like osteoarthritis and for replacing joints destroyed by trauma, artificial joints and the techniques for inserting them were developed beginning in the 1960s, and hundreds of thousands of hips and knees are replaced worldwide every year. Shoulder and finger joints can also be replaced with metal and plastic.

Cochlear implants. Most hearing loss is the result of damage to the hair cells in the inner ear that convert the mechanical energy of sound to electrical energy that can be transmitted through nerves to the brain. Implants replace the function of these hair cells with an external microphone connected to electrodes implanted in the inner ear. The U.S. Food and Drug Administration has approved their use in people over one year old, and although they work best in children who have not yet acquired speech, they have been widely used in adults as well.

Breast implants. The FDA has approved four different kinds. Two companies, Mentor and Allergan, have approvals for both saline- and silicone-gel-filled implants, which are approved for breast reconstruction at any age. For augmentation, the saline are approved for women eighteen and older, and the silicone for women twenty-two and older. Why the different age restrictions? The risks are different. Silicone-gel-filled implants require frequent MRI monitoring to make sure they haven't ruptured without the patient's knowing it; there's no such risk with the saline kind. (The FDA doesn't say what difference the four years make.) There can be other side effects, including additional surgeries, hardening around the implant, and changes in breast and nipple sensation.

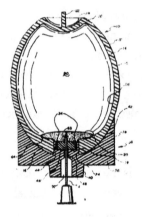

Patent drawing for a testicular implant: we believe the sharp tack is for manufacture only.

Testicular implants. During the 1990s, these purely cosmetic implants were not available in the United States because of doubts about the silicone gel used in them. But now the FDA has approved them once again. Available in a wide range of sizes.

Voice prostheses. A tracheoesophageal voice prosthesis allows people who have had their larynx removed to talk. It involves implanting a valved device that allows air to pass into the esophagus while preventing food or liquid from entering. The wearer exhales through the lungs to produce sound. There are also handheld external devices.

Stents. These are small tubes that can be put in arteries, blood vessels, the ureter, liver ducts, and others to hold the tube open. Probably the most common are the stents used to open coronary arteries that have become blocked.

Thirty People Who Probably Like Having a
Disease Named After Them . . .

"I have Bright's disease, and he has mine," someone once said, probably hoping that a crack like that would get him a seat next to Dorothy Parker at the Algonquin Round Table. The term, which once vaguely described kidney disease, is no longer in use, but all sparkling wittiness aside, doctors and scientists generally consider it a great honor to have a disease named after them. Having one's name on even a bacterium or a virus is a distinction, and virtually an assurance of receiving many large research grants and a lifelong job at an Ivy League university.

Diseases are classified by the World Health Organization in the *International Statistical Classification of Diseases and Related Health Problems*, or *ICD*, which the WHO has been publishing in successive revised editions since 1948. Some specialties also have their own nomenclature authorities. The American Psychiatric Association, for example, publishes the *Diagnostic and Statistical Manual of Mental Disorders*, now in its fourth edition, and thus usually referred to as *DSM-IV*. The classification and naming of diseases dates back to the late nineteenth century, when physicians realized that it was important to record the causes of death more precisely than as a list of casually observed symptoms, which had been the common practice until then.

It is usually, but not always, the person who first describes a disease who gets the honor. There are thousands of syndromes, surgical operations and tools, psychological techniques, tumors and cysts, deformities, and other medical phenomena that have people's names attached to them, and it's sometimes hard to say exactly what is a disease and what isn't. Most would agree, for example, that Alzheimer's is a disease, and so does the *ICD*. But some medical references—*The Merck Manual*, for example—refer to illnesses like Albers-Schönberg's disease, a bone disorder that the *ICD* has never heard of. Often, but not always, rare diseases are the ones that retain the names of their discoverers. The more common diseases eventually get common names. Alzheimer's and Parkinson's are exceptions rather than the rule.

We like the sound of the diseases in this sampling. All of them make the *ICD*; if the WHO considers it a disease, we do, too.

Achilles tendinitis. Inflammation of the Achilles tendon. You may remember the demigod whose mother dipped him in the River Styx in her attempt to make him immortal. Too bad she was holding him by his heel.

Alport's syndrome. A very rare and usually fatal hereditary illness characterized by kidney problems, deafness, and eye abnormalities. Cecil Alport (1880–1959) was a Scottish doctor and a St. Mary's Hospital colleague and friend of Alexander Fleming, the discoverer of penicillin.

Alzheimer's disease. Now considered the most common form of dementia. The German psychiatrist Emil Kraeplin suggested naming the disease after Alois Alzheimer (1864–1915), a fellow psychiatrist and neurologist.

Andersen's disease. An inherited endocrine gland disorder. One of the few diseases named after a woman, Dorothy Hansine Andersen (1901–1963), who described this inherited endocrine gland disorder in 1956. Andersen was also one of the first physicians to identify cystic fibrosis.

Asperger's syndrome. This developmental disorder, typified by abnormal speech and movements, lack of empathy, and repetitive motor activities, may be a type of autism rather than a separate illness. Hans Asperger (1906–1980), an Austrian pediatrician, described it in 1944.

Baló's concentric sclerosis. A brain disease characterized by alternating bands of intact and defective myelin, the sheath that forms around nerve fibers. József Baló (1895–1979) was a widely published Hungarian pathologist who first described the disease in 1926.

Bell's palsy. A paralysis of the facial muscles that usually has a sudden onset and affects only one side of the face. Often the patient cannot control salivation or tearing. Charles Bell (1774–1842) was a British anatomist and surgeon whose most important work was in neurology. He published widely in physiology, neurology, and surgery and had an international reputation as a scientist and physician; at the same time, he was an accomplished artist, producing his own medical illustrations. He was knighted in 1831.

Brucellosis. This is a group of infectious diseases caused by various species of a bacterium called brucella. The disease, and the germ, are named after Sir David Bruce (1855–1931), a famous Scottish infectious disease specialist who worked extensively in Africa. His wife, Mary Elizabeth, was his collaborator. On his deathbed, he is reputed to have said, "Should any notice appear about myself, you must see that my wife gets credit for all the work she has done." So we should presume the disease is named after Lady Bruce as well.

Bruton's disease. Also called agammaglobulinemia, this is a congenital blood disease characterized by susceptibility to bacterial illnesses and joint pain symptoms. Ogden Bruton (1908–2003) discovered the disease in 1951 in a child in the pediatric ward of Walter Reed Army Hospital. The gene associated with the condition also carries his name: Bruton's tyrosine kinase, or Btk.

Charcot-Marie-Tooth disease. Our winner in the Best Name for a Disease contest has nothing to do with teeth. It's an inherited neurological disorder that affects both motor and sensory nerves, causing muscle weakness and deformities in the feet and lower legs. It can be painful, even crippling, but it is rarely fatal. Neurologists Jean-Martin Charcot (1825–1893) and Howard Henry Tooth (1856–1925) were French and English, respectively. See *Marie-Bamberger disease* for Pierre Marie, who got his name attached to several diseases and syndromes.

Cori's disease. The ailment, actually one of a group of diseases called glycogen storage disease, is a rare genetic enzyme deficiency that makes the body deposit abnormal amounts of glycogen in various organs. Husband and wife team Carl (1896–1984) and Gerty Cori (1896–1957) won the Nobel Prize in 1947 for discovering how the process works. There are several variations of the illness, depending on the exact physiological process that explains the abnormal metabolism, and several other people were involved in describing them. So it is sometimes known as Forbes disease, after Gilbert Forbes, who wrote about one type in the early 1950s. A closely related glycogen metabolism disorder is called Hers disease, after a Belgian physiologist named Henri-Géry Hers. Yet another glycogen storage disorder, affecting mainly the liver and kidneys, is called Gierke's disease, after Edgar Otto Conrac von Gierke, who published a paper on it in 1929. The names are sometimes used interchangeably.

Crohn's disease. A chronic bowel disease that can cause inflammation in any part of the digestive tract, but most commonly in the lower part of the small intestine. It can cause painful swelling of the intestine. Gastroenterologist Burrill Crohn (1884–1983) published the first description of "regional enteritis" in 1932.

Cushing's syndrome. A rare hormonal disorder caused by excessive exposure to cortisol. The illness has varied symptoms

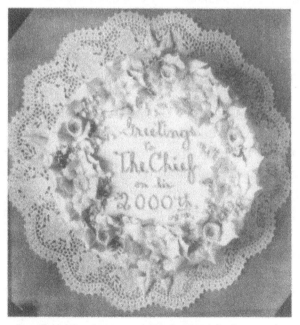

The cake celebrating Dr. Cushing's 2000th brain operation. Really.

including upper body obesity, thin limbs, and bones so weak that ordinary activity can cause fractures. Often called the "father of neurosurgery," Harvey Cushing (1869–1939) was a Johns Hopkins University and later Harvard surgeon.

DiGeorge's syndrome. A congenital abnormality of the thymus gland, associated with facial deformities and frequent infections. Infants usually die from infection, and those who survive are often mentally retarded. It is sometimes genetic, but not always. It is named after an American pediatrician, Angelo DiGeorge (b. 1921).

Duchenne's muscular dystrophy. A muscle disease that usually begins in early childhood. It is almost always fatal before the age of twenty. The French neurologist Guillaume Duchenne (1806–1875) was famous for using electrical stimulation to identify muscle groups in the face, including those responsible for smiles caused by genuine rather than feigned happiness.

Fabry's disease. An inherited metabolic disease that causes impaired kidney function, eye problems, skin lesions, and episodes of fever. It's carried by asymptomatic females, but affects only males and is usually fatal. Johannes Fabry (1860–1930) was a German dermatologist who first described the disease in 1898. It is sometimes called Fabry-Anderson disease after William Anderson, a nineteenth-century British surgeon.

Jakob-Creutzfeldt disease. A very rare fatal brain disease with truly nasty symptoms: stiffness in the limbs, progressive motor and sensory deficits, psychological disturbances, and seizures. The cause of this and related spongiform en-

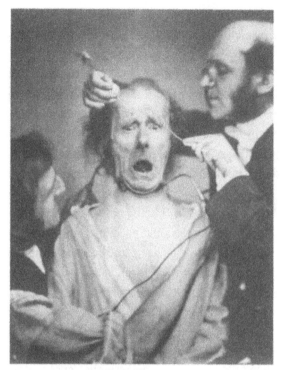

Dr. Duchenne (right) at work.

cephalopathies (such as kuru, also known as "laughing sickness," and mad cow disease, or BSE) is probably a prion, a protein molecule that lacks nucelic acid. Alfons Jakob (1884–1931) and Hans Creutzfeldt (1885–1964) were German neurologists.

Kallmann's syndrome. A congenital disorder of the hypothalamus that causes a deficiency in sex hormone production. It is named for Franz Josef Kallmann (1897–1965), the German-born geneticist who described it in 1944, although the syndrome had been noticed by others earlier. Kallmann immigrated to the United States in 1933, to escape the growing persecution of the Jews.

Marfan's syndrome. An inherited connective tissue disorder that can affect the lungs, eyes, and spinal cord, among other organs. Antoine Marfan (1858–1942), a French pediatrician, first described the disease in 1899. Marfan also has a law named for him: one for diagnosing the course of treatment, based on original onset in childhood, of tuberculosis cases.

Marie-Bamberger disease. This syndrome includes clubbing of the fingers and toes, joint problems, movement disturbances, and often lung cancers and abscesses. It has been known for more than two thousand years—first described by Hippocrates—but Eugen von Bamberger (1858–1921), a Viennese internist, and Pierre Marie (1853–1940), a French neurologist, managed to get their names attached to it. Marie is one of the few to have his name attached to more than one disease—he's the Marie of Marie-Strümpell encephalitis, more often called ankylosing spondylitis, an inflammatory disease of the spine, as well as of the neurological disorder *Charcot-Marie-Tooth disease,* described above.

Niemann-Pick disease. A hereditary metabolic disease similar to Fabry's that has various subtypes with slightly different symptoms. The victims usually die in infancy or early childhood, but there is an adult version as well. Albert Niemann (1880–1921) was a pediatrician and Ludwig Pick (1868–1944) was a pathologist. They found cellular differences between two of the subtypes. Tragically, Niemann died at the age of forty-one and Pick was murdered at seventy-six in a German concentration camp.

Parkinson's disease. James Parkinson (1755–1824), an English surgeon, wrote "An Essay on the Shaking Palsy" in 1817, the first accurate clinical description of the neurological disease that now has his name. Parkinson was not only a doctor but also a radical and outspoken opponent of William Pitt the Younger's government, an enthusiastic defender of the underprivileged, an advocate of universal suffrage, and a member of various secret political societies. He was also the author of popular medical advice books and an advocate for the mentally ill. All this was not enough for Parkinson, however, who then turned his attention to paleontology, publishing an important early work in that field called *Organic Remains of the Former World*, which he illustrated himself. He was a founding member of the Geological Society of London.

Reiter's disease. A rheumatic disease—that is, a disease of the joints—that can also involve the eyes, mouth, skin, and kidneys. Probably caused by an allergic reaction to one of several different bacteria acquired through food or sexual contact. Hans Reiter (1881–1969) was a German kidney specialist. Although he always referred to the disease by his own name, not everyone does, and for good reason: Reiter was a devoted Nazi, and probably participated in medical experimentation with unwilling human subjects. The names Fiessinger and Leroy syndrome are also used, and "reactive arthritis" is the term some journals now prefer.

Sheehan's syndrome. Failure of the function of the pituitary gland following trauma at birth, causing partial or complete loss of function in other glands. It is named for Harold Sheehan (1900–1988), an English pathologist. He was much prouder of his work on the pathology of the kidneys than he was of his description of the syndrome that bears his name.

Steinert's disease. A type of muscular dystrophy that causes muscular wasting, abnormal muscle contractions, cataracts, abnormally small sexual organs, and mental deterioration. It is genetic. The disease was identified in 1909 by Hans Steinert (1875–1911), a German neurologist.

Stokes-Adams disease. A conduction disorder of the heart that causes a temporary blockage of blood flow to the brain. It was first described in the seventeenth century, but the Irish physicians William Stokes (1804–1878) and Robert Adams (1791–1875) described it more systematically. Stokes also got a law named after him: that a muscle sitting above an inflamed membrane will be paralyzed.

Tay-Sachs disease. A genetic lipid storage disorder that causes certain kinds of fats to accumulate in tissues of the brain. Children with the disease die by the age of four. The disease is characterized by a cherry-red spot on the retina, which was noticed and documented in 1894 by British ophthalmologist Warren Tay (1843–1927). Bernard Sachs (1858–1944) was an American neurologist who recognized that the disease is genetic. Sachs was unaware of Tay's work, and it was only later that people realized they were describing the same disease.

Thomsen's disease. A benign inherited muscular disease characterized by slow relaxation of contracted muscles. There is no cure, but symptoms often decline with age. Asmus Thomsen (1815–1896) was a Danish physician who described the disease in himself and his family.

Von Zumbusch's syndrome. A rare form of severe psoriasis that can be life-threatening. Leo Von Zumbusch (1874–1940) was an Austrian dermatologist and syphilis specialist.

Zellweger's syndrome. A rare hereditary disease that has its onset in the womb, characterized by imperfections in the myelin sheath that covers the nerves and by seizures, cataracts, and many abnormalities of bones. It is invariably fatal within a few weeks or months. Hans Zellweger (1909–1990) was a Swiss-born physician who immigrated to America in 1959.

. . . and One Person Who Likely Didn't

Lou Gehrig's disease. Of course no one called it that until the great New York Yankees first baseman Gehrig died of it in 1941, but it's hard to believe that anyone but a doctor would want to have an illness, especially one as tough as this one, named after him. The proper name is amyotrophic lateral sclerosis (ALS), and there are several different types. Some cases are familial; most are not. Although at least one gene mutation is associated with some cases of familial ALS, no one knows exactly what causes it. Some believe it is an autoimmune disease in which the body's immune system attacks normal nerve cells. Researchers have also looked at exposure to toxic substances or infectious agents, but the evidence is not yet strong enough to implicate any of them.

Hometown Germs

While there is no "official" classification of bacteria, there is an organization that approves names for them. The generally agreed-upon authority, the *International Code of Nomenclature of Bacteria*, is published by the American Society for Microbiology. The rules for arriving at a name are a bit complicated, and the society itself admits that "the formal system of naming bacteria appears sometimes tiresome, confusing and even exasperating to the working bacteriologist." Since we strive to be neither tiresome, confusing, nor exasperating, it will be enough to say here that in general a person gets his or her name attached to a bacterium if he or she is the first to publish an article describing it in a peer-reviewed scientific journal.

Viruses have their own naming authority, the International Committee on Taxonomy of Viruses, a unit of the International Union of Microbiological Societies. Its rules are slightly different, but equally complex and obscure, and they are outlined in the *International Code of Virus Classification and Nomenclature*. Publishing first is, as with bacteria, the key to getting your name on a virus.

But then there are names for germs and diseases that aren't the real scientific names but what most people call them. Sometimes having a germ, or the disease that it causes, named after you, your organization, or your geographical location memorializes you for the wrong reasons, lowers real estate values, or makes people think your group or your hometown is full of pestilence. Like these:

Legionnaires' disease. The American Legion held a convention in Philadelphia from July 21 to 24, 1976. Ten thousand people attended. By August 3, fourteen of them had died, apparently from some mysterious disease they had caught at the convention, and twelve others were very sick. A dozen or so deaths among ten thousand people might just be coincidence, but when people as young as thirty-nine are dying, scientists start to wonder. At first they thought the cause might be food poisoning, but the pattern of illness seemed to make that unlikely. Swine flu and poisonous metals were considered. Some doctors decided it was psittacosis, a virus transmitted by contact with bird feathers and droppings—there were plenty of pigeons around to carry it.

On August 3, the *New York Times* reported twenty deaths and 115 hospitalizations—all people who had attended the convention. The autopsies revealed that the participants had died of a severe viral pneumonia. On August 4, two more people died. The next day, one more. By August 8, twenty-seven people were dead. Legionnaires were referring to it as "the illness." On August 11, the *Times* called it "legionnaire's disease," though the name was preceded by "so-called." Who was calling it that before the *Times* did so remains unknown. On August 13, the *Times* dropped the "so-called" and the quotation marks around the name. Barely three weeks after it appeared, and without much of a hint of its cause, the disease had a name. Despite the complaints of some of its members, the American Legion never took an official position against it.

By the way, Legionnaires' disease is caused by a bacterium, which scientists found a few months after the epidemic ended.

Lyme disease. Lyme and Old Lyme are Connecticut towns not far from each other in the southeastern part of the state. Lyme is small—only about two thousand people. The median income for a family in the year 2000 was $82,853, and more

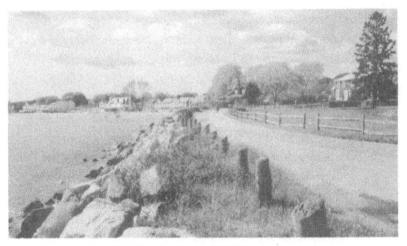

The attractive, tick-friendly shrubs of Old Lyme, Connecticut.

than 98 percent of the people who live there are white. Old Lyme, a popular summer resort, has a permanent population of about 7,500 and shares a school district with Lyme. There's a town called East Lyme, not too far away, which wasn't really involved in the discovery of the disease, but it's stuck with the name anyway.

In 1975, three children in and near Lyme came down with painful, swollen joints. One of them, a nine-year-old girl, had to spend several weeks in a wheelchair. Another had attacks lasting a week or more that came and went several times. Dozens of other cases began accumulating in Lyme, Old Lyme, and nearby East Haddam. Scientists from Yale University figured out that this was a new kind of arthritis, apparently carried by an insect, probably a tick. The scientists had found fifty-one cases by mid-1976, and they were calling it "Lyme arthritis," presumably without consulting the town elders. That term is still used to describe the rheumatic aspects of the illness. The name for the disease as a whole evolved to "Lyme disease," which stuck. East Haddam somehow dodged the bullet.

Lyme has several places listed in the National Register of Historic Places, but the place where the first case of Lyme disease was found is not one of them.

Norwalk virus. The first appearance of Norwalk virus was probably in an outbreak of intestinal disease in 1968 among a group of 232 students at an elementary school in Norwalk, a town in north central Ohio with a population of about 17,000. The germ was definitively identified in 1972 by Dr. Al Kapikan, an employee of the National Institute of Allergy and Infectious Diseases, who examined stool samples from that outbreak.

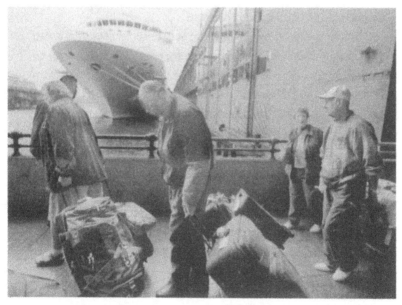

Infection, a cruise ship virus's sweetest reward: passengers disembark from a ship after a suspected Norwalk outbreak.

We think it's worth reiterating that this Norwalk has nothing to do with Norwalk, Connecticut, a much larger and probably better known city of about 83,000 people. Connecticut has enough trouble dealing with the stigma of Lyme disease.

There are periodic outbreaks of Norwalk virus in the United States: 340 people on a cruise ship docked in New York City in September 2003; twenty-eight U.S. Airways passengers flying from Arizona to North Carolina in July 2003; and sixty passengers aboard the Disney cruise ship *Magic* in Florida.

Lassa fever. Lassa fever is an acute viral hemorrhagic fever, endemic in West African countries, and first identified in 1969 in Lassa, Nigeria—a town known, as far as we can tell, for nothing else, and a place so obscure that it can't be found on most maps of Nigeria. But it will ever be remembered in the name of this truly terrible disease.

Lassa is caused by a virus that is carried by rats, and it can be transmitted to humans by contact with their droppings or urine. It can also be transmitted by airborne particles from those droppings. Sometimes people eat the rats, and that's another way the virus can infect humans. You can get a fever, chest pain, sore throat, back pain, cough, abdominal pain, vomiting, diarrhea, conjunctivitis, facial swelling, and mucosal bleeding. You can also suffer hearing loss, tremors, and inflammation of the brain. The death rate is about 1 percent, although getting the disease in the third trimester of pregnancy is almost invariably fatal to the fetus. Nearly a third of those who recover from Lassa fever are left with varying degrees of permanent deafness.

Coxsackie virus. Named for the town of Coxsackie, New York, a small town on the Hudson River where its discoverer,

Gilbert Dalldorf, who worked for the New York State Department of Health, obtained the first fecal specimens that contained the virus. How would you feel if you lived in a town famous for the germs in its feces? No, not too good. So don't laugh.

Coxsackie virus is very contagious, and infection rates are highest among infants and children younger than five years. You get a fever that can last three or four days, and then you usually recover completely and fairly quickly. Some cases are more serious, though, with high fever or fever of unusual duration, or severe sore throat, headache, and difficulty breathing. These cases need the attention of a doctor.

Tularemia. Both the disease and the bacterium that causes it, *Franciscella tularensis*, are named after Tulare County, in central California. You can catch it from animals like rabbits and squirrels, possibly by eating them undercooked, by drinking contaminated water, or by inhalation. The disease is extremely rare—less than one case in a million in the United States between 1990 and 2000. You get a fever, lose your appetite, feel lethargic. It's very incapacitating, but usually you recover. The treatment is antibiotics, either streptomycin, gentamicin, or one of the tetracyclines.

The bacterium is easy to make into an aerosol, and it doesn't take many bacteria to make people ill—which makes it a really neat biological weapon, something that has not gone unnoticed by several countries, including the United States.

SCARED TO DEATH

*No one becomes a good doctor until he
fills a churchyard.*

—SWEDISH PROVERB

Can You Be Scared to Death?

WE'RE ALWAYS CLAIMING THAT WE WERE "SCARED TO
death" or "scared stiff" or sometimes "scared silly" by
something, not to mention having various things "scared
out of us," the words for most of which we wouldn't want to
print in a book like this. These expressions, taken literally,
have been studied, and there's good evidence that people can
indeed die of fright.

An article published in the *Annals of Internal Medicine* describes various stories, some, admittedly, of dubious historic-
ity, of people who dropped dead from strong emotions. The
Roman emperor Nerva (AD 30–98) died in a fit of anger at a
senator who had offended him. The thirteenth-century pope

Innocent IV is said to have died of grief after the overthrow of his army. Some American patriot, it was reported, died of happiness after learning that General Cornwallis's army had been defeated at Yorktown. Well, okay, maybe.

But the study's author, G. L. Engel, also collected, mostly from newspapers, 170 contemporary accounts of sudden death attributed to disruptive life events. He classified them into seven categories: death of someone close; the threat of a death of someone close; during grief; during mourning or on an anniversary; on losing status or self-esteem; on threat of injury; after the threat is over. He added one more, a case, you might say, of dying of happiness: death upon a reunion, or happy ending. Most of the deaths, he says, occurred within an hour of the event reported.

There are plausible mechanisms that can explain why strong emotions can result in death. An article titled "The Brain-Heart Connection" outlines some of the theory: that cardiac problems can be caused by what the author, Dr. Martin Samuels, calls a "generalized autonomic storm, which occurs as a result of a life-threatening stressor." Essentially, the nervous system can be stimulated in such a way as to cause a heart attack and death. Although you obviously can't experiment with humans, there's plenty of experimental evidence in animals to show that this can happen, specifically by stimulating the part of the brain called the hypothalamus, which causes cardiac lesions and death.

Another study looked at 3,015 people aged seventy to seventy-nine to see whether those who were more anxious were more likely to die. They found, surprisingly, a racial difference: anxiety was a predictor of death in black people, but not in whites.

Can You Be Scared Stiff?

Some animals get scared stiff, in the sense that they become immobilized in order to hide from a threat. More or less the same thing can happen to people. Catatonia—a paralysis that has no apparent physical cause—is a well-known psychiatric disorder, and it can be provoked by fear.

A 2004 study suggests that the reaction originally served the same purpose it does in some animals: protection from the threat of being eaten by another animal. But now it is provoked, inappropriately, by other kinds of fear, anxiety, or feelings of imminent doom, real or imagined.

People who experience catatonia report a subjective state of extreme anxiety, and the disorder can be treated with benzodiazepines (anti-anxiety drugs). In some cases the medicine works within a matter of minutes.

There are reports of fatal catatonia, with the deaths arising from kidney failure, cardiovascular collapse, or cardiac arrhythmias. One study reported that almost 80 percent of autopsies in catatonia found no medical cause of death.

Catching Our Breath

While boys are more likely than girls to be diagnosed with asthma during childhood, women are more likely than men to have asthma in adulthood.

American Adults with Asthma

"Have you ever been told by a doctor or other health professional that you had asthma?"

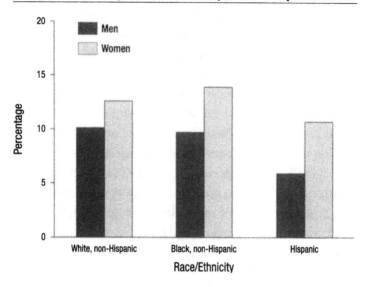

Can You Die of a Broken Heart?

Obviously, yes, if you mean can you die because your heart gets broken in the sense that it stops working properly. People die of that kind of broken heart every day. But usually the phrase is used to describe dying because of strong emotions, especially those brought on by a failed romance. That's tricky.

Acute stress can cause heart failure, and a failed romance may be stressful enough to do it. So that's dying of a broken heart, in a sense. But of course sometimes people under stress already have heart disease, so whether the stress caused the fatal heart disease is not clear. Yet there is a syndrome called acute stress cardiomyopathy, which looks a lot like a heart attack but isn't one, and is caused by stressful events. An article published in 2008 describes the syndrome.

Apparently the disorder has many of the same symptoms as a heart attack—chest pain, an irregular electrocardiogram, elevated cardiac enzymes, and abnormal motion in the left ventricle of the heart. But it's not a heart attack.

Usually these are people without evidence of cardiac disease who come into the hospital after acute emotional or physical stress. The most common emotional triggers are grief (the death of a loved one, for example) or fear (being robbed at gunpoint or being involved in a car accident).

The syndrome was first noted in Japan but has been seen in people all over the world. Most of the patients, as many as 90 percent, are women, and they're usually older than sixty-two. Risk factors for coronary illness are common, with half of the victims having high blood pressure, and about a third with high lipid levels. About 11 percent have a history of heart disease in their families.

Treatment is usually just supportive—you give the patients some of the same medicines used in treating heart attacks and they gradually get better. But a few—probably less than 3 percent—die. When researchers looked at how the survivors did after the incident, their death rate was no greater than that of other people their own age and sex.

What's happening here? Are the people who die of acute stress cardiomyopathy dying of a broken heart? The stress makes plasma catecholamine levels rise—much more so than in people who are having true heart attacks. Catecholamines are a group of chemicals that includes epinephrine, which can cause various physiological effects associated with stress. Exactly how these chemical changes result in abnormal heart function is not clear. But if grief, for example, causes a series of chemical reactions in the body that lead to heart abnormalities, and the heart abnormalities lead to death, then maybe dying of a broken heart is a real phenomenon, and not just a metaphor.

Good for the Heart

Finally, things are looking up. Heart disease is still the leading cause of death in the United States, but fewer people are getting it.

Hospitalization Rates for Coronary Atherosclerosis and Heart Attacks

Per 10,000 population

The Top Ten Killers

When people think of scary diseases, their minds often wander to spectacular and exotic infections like avian flu, dengue fever, or Ebola. These are serious and growing problems in some parts of the world, but they're unlikely to affect the average American, who doesn't usually travel to the places where they are endemic. (Of course, this doesn't mean they won't become a problem in the future—possibly the near future. With the right combination of conditions, diseases can spread rapidly over the globe.) And people often fear the sort of diseases you "catch": Yikes! Germs! Well, germs can cause some unpleasant problems, up to and including death. But among the top killers of Americans, only two are diseases you "catch." Developing the others is more complicated than that.

The ten most deadly diseases in the United States don't always get the most publicity, either. Breast cancer, for example, is certainly a serious problem, but lung cancer kills more women, and so do heart disease and stroke.

Here are the diseases Americans should worry about (the final 2005 figures were published in 2008):

1. Heart disease. It's a preventable disease, at least partly, but it killed 652,091 people in 2005. More than one-quarter of women die from diseases of the heart, but according to a survey done by the CDC, only 13 percent of women think that heart disease is their greatest health threat. And it's not just old women who die of heart disease. It's the third leading cause of death among women aged twenty-five to forty-four and the second leading cause among those forty-five to sixty-four.

2. Cancer. 559,312 people died of some kind of cancer in 2005, even though cancer deaths overall have been declining. From 2002 through 2004, they declined at a rate of 2.1 percent a year.

The three leading causes of cancer death in men were lung, prostate, and colorectal cancer.

If you're a woman, the kind of cancer you should be most

worried about is lung cancer—it is the number one cancer killer of women, and it kills about twice as many women as breast cancer. The American Cancer Society estimates that in 2008 lung cancer killed about 70,000 women while breast cancer killed about 40,000. Maybe lung cancer should have a ribbon, too, but for some reason lung cancer victims don't inspire the same kind of solidarity that breast cancer victims do. Maybe it's because most lung cancer is caused by an avoidable behavior: smoking.

3. *Stroke.* Strokes happen when the blood supply to the brain is blocked or when a blood vessel in the brain bursts. About 700,000 people have a stroke every year, according to the CDC, and 75 percent of them are older than sixty-five. If you survive a stroke, you can have anything from no disability at all to an inability to speak, emotional problems, or paralysis. In 2005, 143,579 had strokes and died, making it the third leading cause of death. High blood pressure, smoking, excessive drinking, diabetes, and heart disease are risk factors that can be controlled.

4. *Chronic lower respiratory disease.* This is actually a group of related diseases including chronic obstructive pulmonary disease, emphysema, chronic bronchitis, and other lung diseases. The primary cause of these diseases is cigarette smoking, so this is yet another preventable illness. CLRD killed 130,933 in 2005, and of these 68,498 were women.

5. *Diabetes.* About 24 million Americans have diabetes, and it's a major cause of kidney failure, amputations, blindness, heart disease, stroke, and premature death. It accounts for more than 40 percent of cases of kidney failure and 60 percent of nontraumatic limb amputations. It's the leading cause of blindness in people ages twenty to seventy-four.

What's more, the disease is becoming more common. For a girl born in 2000, the lifetime risk of getting diabetes is about 33 percent; for a boy, it's even higher, around 38 percent. In 2005, 75,119 death certificates listed diabetes as the underlying cause of death.

6. *Alzheimer's disease.* Age and family history are the main risk factors for this incurable disease, and no one knows what causes it. About 5 million people have it, and 71,599 died from it in 2005.

7. *Influenza and pneumonia.* Of the 63,001 people who died of the flu, 88 percent were over sixty-five. But it also killed 653 people under age twenty-five, including 265 babies under one year old. The moral? Follow the CDC's recommendation for flu shots: children six months to nineteen years, pregnant women, people over age fifty, people with certain medical conditions, and anyone who has contact with people at risk for the flu should get a flu vaccine every year. This includes most of you, so what are you waiting for?

8. *Kidney disease.* The 43,901 total for kidney disease deaths includes a group of kidney ailments—nephritis, acute nephritic syndrome, renal failure, and other disorders—but it does not include the more than 12,000 people who died of kidney cancer.

9. *Septicemia.* Septicemia is caused by bacteria spreading in the blood, and it's one of only two infectious diseases in the top-ten killer list. In 2005, 34,136 people died of it.

10. *Chronic liver disease.* Chronic liver disease, mostly caused by excessive drinking and hepatitis, killed 27,530 in 2005. The

diagnosis includes several different conditions, diseases, and infections that affect the liver, some of which are preventable or treatable. Alcoholic liver disease accounted for 12,928 of these deaths, all of which, presumably, were preventable.

What Are You Most Likely to Die Of?

It depends on how old you are. If you're fifteen to twenty-four years old, you're more likely to die in an accident than by all the other causes of death combined. And the most likely way you'll go to your reward will be in a car crash, twice as common as any other kind of accident. If that doesn't kill you, the second most likely way to die is getting murdered. Other accidents are third, and suicide is fourth. You have to go down the list to fifth place before a disease kicks in—cancer.

By the time you're between twenty-five and forty-four, you die in car accidents at a much lower rate—about two-thirds the rate of younger people. But accidents of some kind are still your biggest risk, with cancer coming in second. Now heart disease places third for this age group, and suicide is still fourth. Homicide is fifth, and then HIV.

When you hit the forty-five to sixty-four age group, it's cancer that's the number one killer, followed by heart disease. Accidents come in a distant third, and people are becoming better drivers—they die in car accidents at a slightly lower rate than the younger age bands.

After age sixty-five, heart disease ranks number one, followed by cancer; cerebrovascular disease is third, then chronic lung disease; Alzheimer's comes in fifth, with pneumonia and diabetes pulling in sixth and seventh. Accidents are eighth, and although the car accident death rate goes up a little for this group, it doesn't nearly reach the level for those under twenty-five, who are by far the worst drivers on the road.

Death by Accident

The CDC says that more than 99 percent of deaths occurring in the United States are registered—that is, death certificates are signed and filed. It is these death certificates from all fifty states and the District of Columbia that the CDC relies on for their numbers.

CDC statistics are presented in accordance with World Health Organization regulations, which specify and classify causes of death. Sometimes more than one cause of death is entered on a death certificate, in which case the CDC determines the underlying cause by the sequence of conditions in the certificate and other rules and provisions of the WHO. It is that underlying cause that they use in their tabulations.

The CDC lists alcohol deaths separately when they're caused by behavioral disorders due to alcohol use, degeneration of the nervous system, accidental exposure to alcohol, and other diseases and conditions caused by alcohol abuse. The deaths below don't include any of those, but they certainly include lots of people who were drunk when they died.

In 2006, 117,809 Americans were killed in accidents. Of these, almost 40 percent died in car accidents, the largest number for any cause, and more than twice as many as the second most common cause of accidental death, poisoning. Other transport accidents, including water, air, space, and unspecified, accounted for 1,852 deaths. Almost 3,500 people drowned.

There are lots of accidental ways to die, and some are more common than others. But not everyone understands what's likely to happen and what isn't. For example, many people are aware that you can die from carbon monoxide poisoning—in New York City, a law requires every dwelling to have a carbon monoxide detector. And according to the CDC, an average of 439 people a year nationwide died from non-fire-related CO poisoning from 1999 to 2004. That's a lot, especially if you or someone you know is one of them. But it is not a lot compared to other, less publicized ways of dying—like falling down, which kills almost 20,000 people a year, or medical and surgical accidents, which kill about 2,500.

The CDC reports the following mayhem for 2006:

Total Accidental Deaths: 117,748

Transport accidents: 47,601
  Motor vehicle accidents: 44,572
  Water, air, space, and other unspecified transport
    accidents: 1,852
  Other unspecified land transport: 1,177

Nontransport accidents: 70,147
  Falls: 20,533
  Accidental discharge of firearms: 777
  Accidental drowning: 3,483
  Exposure to smoke and flames: 3,066
  Poisoning: 24,702
  Other unspecified accidents: 17,586

From 1999 to 2004, there were fewer deaths from drowning and burning, while deaths by poisoning and in motorcycle accidents each increased by more than 60 percent.

Change in Death Rates for Various Accidents

Between 1994 and 2004, there were fewer deaths from drowning and burning, while deaths by poisoning and in motorcycle accidents each increased by more than 60 percent.

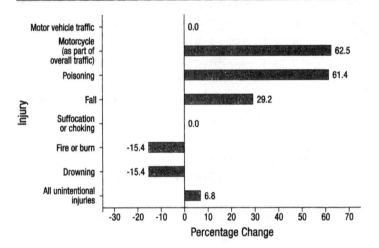

Of course, some deaths aren't exactly accidents, but they're not exactly natural either:

Legal intervention: 411
This includes injuries inflicted by police or other law-enforcement agents in the course of performing their legal duty.

Complications of medical and surgical care: 2,492
This includes surgical accidents and errors in drug administration.

Events of undetermined intent: 4,492
We don't know what this includes. Which is the point.

Which Is More Common, Suicide or Homicide?

Suicide—and it's not even close. In 2005, there were 33,637 suicides in the United States and 18,124 homicides.

The older you are, the less likely you will be murdered and the more likely you will commit suicide. Fifteen- to twenty-four-year-olds are the only group in which fewer people commit suicide than are murdered. In 2005, there were 5,359 murders and 4,139 suicides in this age group (both of which are still lower than the number who died in a car accident—10,830 that year). For all adults over age eighteen, the rate of suicide is almost twice the rate of homicide. By age group, the highest rate of suicide is in people over seventy-five years old, who are about eight times as likely to kill themselves as they are to be murdered.

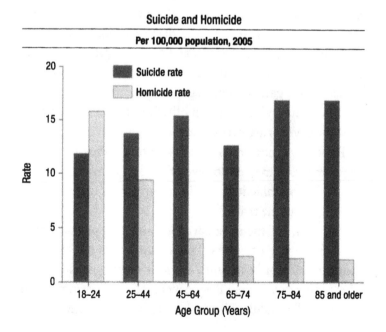

Suicide and Homicide

Per 100,000 population, 2005

Of all suicides, 17,002—almost exactly half—of the people killed themselves with guns. In homicides, guns were the weapon in 12,352, about 68 percent.

When someone gets shot to death, it's usually pretty easy to tell whether it was a suicide, a homicide, or an accident. But when people get poisoned it's much less simple. In 2005, there were 32,691 deaths caused by poison. Authorities determined that most of them—about 72 percent—were accidents, and about 18 percent were suicides. The other 10 percent? They couldn't say.

Plants That Can Kill You

Most plants contain poisons. That's because plants can't run away from animals that want to eat them. Their only defense is to taste bad, or make the animal who eats them sick, even sick unto death. There are more than seven hundred species of plants in the United States and Canada that have caused illness or death in humans, and many are commonly found in homes, flower gardens, and vegetable gardens, and as decorative plants around houses. And that's not even counting the wild ones, which are everywhere.

Poison ivy, poison oak, poison sumac—they're just the beginning, and they're not even that dangerous. An oozing rash and unbearable itching? That's nothing. No, we're talking here about the real killers.

And some of the most harmless-sounding plants contain some of the worst poisons. Take castor beans, the source of castor oil. Castor beans are a member of the genus Ricinus, which gives you a hint. They contain so much ricin that one bean can kill an adult. The ricin has to be removed in order to

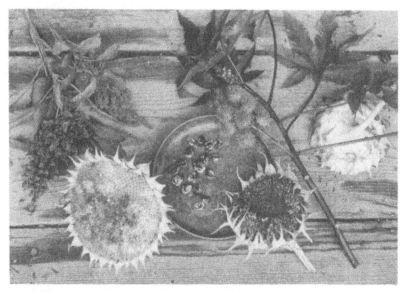

The pretty and pretty deadly castor plant.

make castor oil. The plant is kind of pretty and is widely used as an ornamental.

Some of the most deadly plants seem perfectly ordinary. English yew, daffodils, oleander, and rhododendron have such nice names you'd hardly believe they could kill you if you happen to ingest too much or the wrong part. Yews, a kind of conifer commonly used in landscaping, produce pretty red berries, which are the only part of the plant that isn't poisonous. Eat any other part and you're likely to fall into convulsions and become paralyzed. With daffodils, it's the bulbs that are poisonous—not that you're likely to be tempted to eat one. Oleander, with its pretty white flowers, is very popular as a decorative shrub. It's full of poisons—nerioside, oleandroside, saponins—and it's a common reason for fatalities among horses and other livestock. Rhododendrons and the closely related azalea come in lots of pretty colors and with something called andromedotoxin that can make you nauseated, paralyzed, and dead. The berries produced by lily of the valley plants in the fall are poisonous. They grow close to the ground, so watch your children: they might decide to try them to see if they taste good.

Does anyone have to wonder whether plants named chokecherry, nightshade, snakeroot, and strychnine tree are good for you? (They're not.)

There are about two thousand plant species that contain prussic acid, better known as cyanide. Neither animals nor humans would be tempted to eat most of them, so they don't commonly present any danger. The stones of cherries, plums, peaches, and the fruit of the bitter almond tree are a good source of cyanide, and it's fortunate that they're not appetizing. Ancient Romans and Egyptians, however, used peach pits to execute people. A fraction of an ounce of cyanide will kill a grown man, which we assume is why spies carry the stuff in those little capsules in case they're captured. At least they do in the movies.

Some plants that we commonly eat are actually poisonous if eaten in large enough quantities. All parts of the sunflower, for example, are called "slightly toxic" by the U.S. Department of Agriculture, but you'd have to eat an awful lot of sunflower seeds before you felt any effects. Rhubarb pie, made with the stems, is tasty, but the leaves have various poisonous substances in them. Admittedly, you'd have to eat about ten pounds of them to get enough to kill you, but still.

Death by Natural Disaster

Lightning, floods, snowstorms, tornadoes, hurricanes, wild-fires, droughts, earthquakes—it's a jungle out there. Well, okay, it's not a jungle, but there are plenty of natural disasters waiting to do you in.

Your nightmares about natural disasters are probably ex-aggerated, but let's face it: these things happen, and you read about them in the paper every day. So where can you live to avoid them? In the United States, almost no place is safe from the wrath of nature, but some places are safer than others.

Researchers have created what amounts to a death map of the United States, using data on natural disasters going back almost forty years and plotting them geographically.

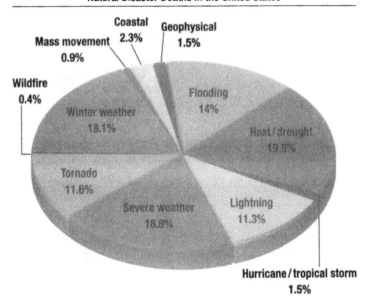

Natural Disaster Deaths in the United States

Coastal 2.3%
Mass movement 0.9%
Geophysical 1.5%
Wildfire 0.4%
Flooding 14%
Winter weather 18.1%
Heat/drought 19.6%
Tornado 11.6%
Severe weather 18.8%
Lightning 11.3%
Hurricane/tropical storm 1.5%

There are, of course, regional differences in the kind of natural disaster you're exposed to. Tornadoes occur in the Midwest; coastal flooding doesn't. But some regions are more severely affected than others. In general, researchers found, there is a greater risk of death along the hurricane coasts, in rural areas, and in the South—those are the places where population growth coincides with frequency of natural disasters. The researchers also found clusters of high mortality in the lower Mississippi Valley, the upper Great Plains, the Mountain West, western Texas, and the panhandle of Florida.

Which natural events are the most dangerous? Maybe not the ones you think. Hurricanes, earthquakes, and wildfires make for great television, but the real killer is plain bad weather, hot and cold. These, combined with storms and floods, cause about 85 percent of deaths. Lightning, hurricanes, tornadoes, and earthquakes are certainly no fun, but they're not the most dangerous things nature throws at us.

11

GRAY MATTER

The doctor should be opaque to his patients and, like a mirror, should show them nothing but what is shown to him.

—SIGMUND FREUD (1856–1939)

Why Do We Need Sleep?

SLEEP HAS BEEN WIDELY STUDIED, AND WE'VE LEARNED A lot about it. Scientists have measured sleeping people's brains using electroencephalographs, and they understand the way sleep is organized. A normal night begins with a period of non-rapid-eye-movement (NREM) sleep, sleep in which your eyes don't move. You then go through four stages, each deeper and less subject to arousal, an effect that can be seen on an EEG as slower waves. In about forty-five minutes, you've cycled through all four stages. Stages 3 and 4, called slow-wave sleep, dominate for the first third of the night, adding up to about 15 to 25 percent of your sleep time.

Then there are the well-known REM (rapid-eye-movement) periods of sleep. The first REM period starts about two hours into your night, and then you alternate between REM and NREM sleep periods in cycles of about an hour and a half.

Think you're getting less sleep than you used to? A lot of people think they are.

You'll also get less stage 3 and 4 slow-wave sleep as you age. The amount most people get is most intense during childhood, decreases at puberty, and declines gradually throughout life. In healthy older people, it can be absent entirely. REM sleep goes through a different evolution. It makes up about half of an infant's sleep time, then falls off sharply over the first year of life. After that, the amount of REM sleep you get remains fairly constant throughout life.

Where sleep happens—in the biological sense—isn't entirely clear. Experiments in animals suggest that certain parts of the brain control sleep—the medullary reticular formation, the thalamus, the basal forebrain. Usually in REM sleep, the muscles are paralyzed, and a lesion on the pons, another part of the brain, can cause people to lose this paralysis. So the pons apparently has something to do with sleep, too. One theory suggests that there is a group of neurons extending from the brain stem that generate the capacity for sleep and wakefulness, because some of them seem to be selectively activated during sleep. But there's no general agreement about these things.

Scientists believe that there are some neurotransmitters associated with sleep, and the effects of various chemicals on sleep and wakefulness have been widely studied. They've done experiments with humans to identify circadian rhythms as well as the various kinds of physiological changes that

Getting Less than Six Hours of Sleep a Night

The National Sleep Foundation recommends that adults get seven to nine hours of sleep each night.

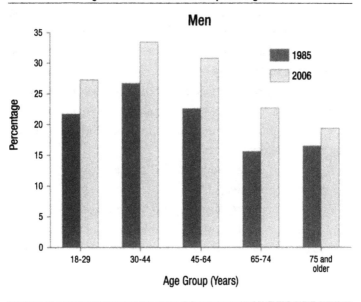

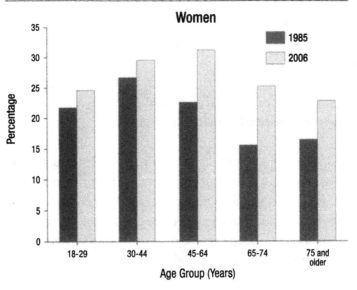

happen—decrease in blood pressure and heart rate, secretion of growth hormone, secretion of the luteinizing hormone during sleep in puberty, and inhibition of it in sleep in adult women in the early phase of the menstrual cycle. They discovered that melatonin is secreted from the pineal gland during sleep. Body temperature drops during sleep and in REM sleep; there's almost no response to changes in temperature at all. Extreme ambient temperatures prevent REM sleep, which may act as a safety feature.

Researchers have also learned a lot about the diseases associated with poor sleep.

But as compelling, obvious, and universal as the need for sleep is, no one really knows why we need it. For now, we'll have to be content with the idea that we need to sleep because we just do.

Ten Psychiatric Illnesses You've Hopefully Never Heard Of

All of these are psychiatric diseases included in the *Diagnostic and Statistical Manual of Mental Disorders*, fourth edition (familiarly referred to as the *DSM-IV*):

Rett's disorder. A rare disease of infancy, reported only in girls, in which a child appears normal for the first five months of life, after which time her head growth slows. Between the ages of five and thirty months, the child loses the ability to move her hands properly and develops a kind of stereotyped movement that resembles hand-washing. Language development is also severely affected.

Rumination disorder. Another disorder of young childhood in which partially digested food is regurgitated into the mouth without any apparent choking or expressions of disgust (on the contrary, they appear to gain some satisfaction from the process), then is either spit out or, more commonly, rechewed and reswallowed. The symptoms are not due to a gastrointestinal problem of any kind. Weight loss and even death can result.

Selective mutism. Children with this disorder persistently fail to speak in certain situations where speaking is expected, such as in school or with playmates. To get this diagnosis, the failure to speak must not be associated with another speech defect (such as stuttering) or with general shyness about new situations. Sometimes children with this disorder communicate with grunts, nodding, or gestures, or in an altered voice.

Caffeine intoxication. You don't need fifteen cups of coffee to become a head case. For people who have this problem, even a hundred milligrams a day—hardly more than a cup of coffee—can result in restlessness, nervousness, overexcitement, insomnia, flushed face, increased urine production, muscle twitching, rambling thoughts, rapid heartbeat, and stomach problems. To get this diagnosis, the patient has to be troubled by the symptoms. If you're drinking all that coffee in order to feel this way—you know who you are—then you don't have a mental disorder.

Nicotine dependence. Yes, it's a psychiatric illness. People dependent on nicotine keep smoking even when it means changing their social life (not flying in airplanes, avoiding social occasions where smoking is prohibited, etc.) and even when they are suffering smoking-related diseases such as bronchitis, chronic obstructive lung disease, or lung cancer.

Dissociative fugue. The main symptom is sudden, unplanned, and unexpected travel away from home with the inability to remember where you went or what you were doing. Sometimes people are confused about their identity, or invent a new identity, when suffering from the illness. People who have this problem don't seem ill during an episode, and usually don't attract much attention. Some even engage in complex social activities under a new personality that seems completely normal.

Frotteurism. Touching or rubbing up against people who don't consent to being touched or rubbed. It usually happens in crowds, where a person, typically a man between the ages of fifteen and twenty-five, rubs his genitalia against the victim's thighs or buttocks, or fondles her. It usually involves a fantasy of having a real and normal intimate relationship with the woman.

Trichotillomania. The recurrent pulling out of one's own hair, resulting in noticeable hair loss. People with the disorder try to resist the action, but the increasing sense of tension they feel is only relieved by engaging in it. The action produces not only relief from the tension, but a sense of pleasure and gratification as well.

Intermittent explosive disorder. Repeated explosive episodes of aggression that result in destruction of property or serious acts of physical assault. The degree of aggressiveness displayed is completely out of proportion to the provocation. The person may say that the acts are the result of "spells" or "attacks" in which the explosive behavior is followed by a sense of relief. Often, the person later feels significant remorse or embarrassment about the incident. You have to be otherwise psychologically healthy to get this diagnosis—you don't get it if the rages are the result of drug use or some other disease.

Neuroleptic-induced acute akathisia. This is among several conditions caused by taking drugs to treat another psychiatric illness. The person is fidgety, rocks back and forth, paces, can't sit still. The disorder develops within a short time after starting or increasing the dose of antipsychotic medicines like Haldol, Clozaril, Risperdal, and Zyprexa.

Left- and Right-Handedness

It may be that one of the reasons handedness is so mysterious is that no one really agrees on definitions. Some people think that if you write with your left hand you're a lefty and if you write with your right hand you're a righty. Others think that a third category, for ambidexterity, ought to be included. But "ambidexterity" itself is a vague term. Everyone knows that there are baseball players who throw righty and bat lefty. Some people play tennis righty, but golf lefty. There are a few very rare cases of people who can write equally well with either hand—we once met a woman who chose to sign her name with whichever hand was nearer to an available pen. She was a righty in almost all other respects except that she played pool lefty! This kind of phenomenon is why some people believe that handedness should be considered along a continuum. It's easy enough to find people who are a little, somewhat, more or less, pretty much, very, mostly, or completely right- or left-handed, and just as easy to invent even more categories in between those.

So how many people are right-handed and how many left-handed? Knowing what we do about the possibilities and variations, the question seems a little simple-minded. In fact, the only way most researchers can determine who's a lefty is to ask. But asking doesn't necessarily produce clear answers. There's no way to sort out the categories, so the design of a questionnaire becomes an exercise in subjectivity. If you have only two or three categories—for example, right-handed, left-handed, or ambidextrous—then depending on how you ask the questions, you're going to get widely varying results. Many people just don't fit the categories.

Looking for a physiological indication of handedness is just as frustrating. The human brain has two hemispheres, left and right. They look alike, and in most respects, but not all, they are alike. Some functions are controlled by the right hemisphere, others by the left. For example, in most people, language is controlled by a part of the left hemisphere. Most, but not all. To figure out where language is controlled in any individual, you would have to do a fairly complex piece of brain surgery, so of course this is impossible. But by examining people who are brain-injured, researchers have concluded that somewhere between 70 percent and 95 percent of people have their language center in the left hemisphere.

Paul Broca, the nineteenth-century discoverer of the language center of the brain, thought that people who had their language center in the left hemisphere were right-handed and those who had it in the right were left-handed. That would be neat, if it were true. But it's not. Most left-handers have their language center on the left, too.

No one knows for sure whether handedness is inherited, but some believe it is. Still, two left-handed parents can give birth to right-handed children, and vice versa. There are interesting theories about the genetics of handedness, but no one has ever actually found a gene for it. To make things even more confusing, one recent twin study found a very small genetic effect on handedness in male twins, none in female twins, and none on footedness in either sex. They concluded that there must be environmental factors at work, but when they looked for those they could find them only in females, not males.

One group of researchers tried to find some data about the environmental causes of handedness by looking at old movies. They watched eight hundred short films made from 1900 to 1906 to try to spot people waving with their left hands, presumably a mark of being left-handed. They found 391 waving people, 61 of whom were waving lefty. Then they compared this to a sample of 391 contemporary films of people waving and found 95 of them sticking up their left arms. Conclusion? Left-handedness declined in Victorian England because of social and school pressures and the rise of industrial tools. Some may find this study interesting; others may even find it convincing. Will we be forgiven if we view it as an illustration of how desperate researchers are to find a way to resolve this question?

The practical problems of being left-handed in a right-handed world are familiar to all lefties. Try finding a pair of scissors usable with your left hand. For Christmas, give a digital camera to your favorite lefty—one with the shutter button on the left instead of the right, if you can find one.

How about one of those can openers that operates by squeezing the handles with one hand and operating the crank with the other. Are any of these gadgets designed so that a lefty can use one comfortably? Not that we've ever seen. We once asked a left-handed surgeon how he managed. Not comfortably, it turns out. Most surgical tools with which handedness is a factor are designed for righties. Almost all instructional videos—essential for a surgeon's education—show right-handed surgeons at work. A lefty surgeon has to imagine everything switched around in order to figure out how to do an operation.

It may be that men are better at telling their right hands from their left than women. Figuring out which is which depends on having an asymmetrical brain—that is, the left half has to be different in some way from the right half. Men's brains tend to be more asymmetrical.

There's plenty of half-baked talk in the popular press about being "right-brained" and "left-brained," and how left-brained people are more creative than right-brained people (or is it the other way around?) and how you can perfect either left-brainedness or right-brainedness and change your personality and improve your life by doing so. Most of this is just jabber. Little is actually known about the effect of either brain lateralization or handedness on intellect or personality. A quick Google search will produce long lists of famous people who were left-handed. The Boston Strangler and Jack the Ripper were both lefties. So were Helen Keller, Ronald Reagan, and Julius Caesar. Robert McNamara and Fidel Castro are lefties, too. And so is Barack Obama. So what? This, finally, is a question about handedness that we can answer definitively, and the answer is: so nothing.

So How Come They Can't Do Long Division?

You may have thought that kids missed school a lot, but it's not so. According to the CDC, 29 percent of kids never missed a single day of school in 2006. Fifty-six percent missed one to five days, 10 percent missed six to ten days, and only 5 percent missed as much as eleven days of school or more.

Why Teenagers Act Nuts

"What were you thinking?" may be among the most common questions parents ask their teenage children when faced with their irrational or apparently self-destructive behavior. Researchers have asked the same question. They've come up with some answers, but they're not always clear or definitive.

Some people think that they do crazy things because they don't have enough information, that there's something they can be taught that would make them more informed and alter their attitudes. But most efforts of this kind don't work. Adolescents are perfectly capable of learning about safe sex and safe driving. The reasoning skills of a sixteen-year-old are just as good as an adult's. They understand risk just as well as grown-ups do. But understanding doesn't change their behavior. They drive too fast and have unprotected sex anyway.

Younger kids and adults don't take the same kinds of risks. Most researchers believe that there is something about adolescents' developing brains that makes them different from the brains of the rest of us. The problem, at least one researcher believes, is that adolescents' logical skills develop by the age of fifteen or so, but psychosocial maturity—the control of impulses and emotions, understanding the advantages of delayed gratification, resistance to peer pressure—takes longer, and is sometimes not fully developed until age twenty-five or older. Without these skills, it's easy to make very bad decisions.

This theory finds some support in neurology. Apparently there are two different brain networks involved. The first is sensitive to social and emotional stimuli, and the hormonal changes of puberty alter this network. It is located in the interior sections of the brain, which include the amygdala, the ventral striatum, the orbitofrontal cortex, and some other areas. The part of the brain that controls functions like planning and thinking ahead—located mainly in the outer regions of the brain—matures more slowly. The two areas compete when it comes to risk taking, and in adolescents the parts that control planning and thinking tend to come out on the losing end until their development has a chance to catch up.

Scientists have actually managed to see this, as it were, in action. The researchers connected adults and adolescents to functional MRI machines, which can track activity in the brain. When they asked them questions like "Is it dangerous to set your hair on fire?" adolescents consistently took longer to respond and activated a narrower part of their brains than adults. This didn't happen when they were asked questions about activities that are not dangerous—eating salad, for example. The kids were able to be very adult and decisive about health food. Setting their hair on fire, on the other hand, gets them wondering.

12

AN APPENDIX

Is the Appendix Really Useless?

WHILE YOU CAN CERTAINLY GET BY WITHOUT THE APPENdix, that doesn't mean it's useless. (Just like the endnotes.) The appendix is the first organ that comes to mind when you think of something inside you that you could just as easily do without. It seems to do nothing until it starts causing trouble—pain, bad infection sometimes, and often an unpleasant operation to get rid of it. But recent research suggests that it may have—or at least had, at one time—an important function.

The appendix is a tube at the end of the ascending colon, a little pouch with a very small opening into the rest of the large intestine, and few species besides humans have one. Some have assumed that it's some kind of evolutionary leftover, but there isn't much evidence that our ancestors had one either.

In 2007, researchers published a novel theory: in times of trouble with diarrheal illnesses, which flush the system of all microorganisms, including the helpful ones, the appendix might serve as a hideout in the body for beneficial organisms until infection passes. After the illness wanes, the gut would be repopulated with these essential bacteria that aid in digestion and fight infection. The scientists stress that this is a deduction, based not on any experimental proof but on new information about the way beneficial microbes live in biofilms, outside the cells, in the human digestive tract. With improvements in sanitation and water supply, this function of the appendix may now be mostly redundant, leaving the impression that the organ is useless.

Tonsils and adenoids are lymphoid tissue, and generally speaking, lymph tissue functions in antibody production. Producing antibodies is usually a good thing—they fight infection. So presumably tonsils and adenoids protect against germs, and the organs are conveniently located in our throats, an obvious place for germs to get in. But people seem to do fine without their tonsils and adenoids, so their function remains a bit of a mystery.

Tonsillectomy, or adenotonsillectomy (the operation in which a doctor removes both the tonsils and the adenoids, lymph tissue in the back of the nose), was at one time a fairly routine operation for kids who suffered from frequent sore throats. Now, not so much. A large review of randomized, controlled trials of tonsillectomy or adenotonsillectomy found that the operations have, at best, mixed results. It will certainly prevent "tonsillitis"—you can't have inflammation in an organ that isn't there—and it may give modest relief to some kids. But most kids start to get fewer sore throats as they get older, without surgery. The average patient will have seventeen rather than twenty-two days of sore throats—and some of those seventeen sore-throat days will be caused by the surgery itself. There's wide variability, of course, and each child is different, but for most children the benefits probably do not outweigh the risks.

There's also the "useless" spleen. Most vertebrates other than humans don't have tonsils or an appendix, but all of them have a spleen. It has two identified functions: to help filter waste material from the blood, including bacteria and unneeded or damaged red blood cells, and to fight infection by producing lymphocytes. The spleen has a clever filtering and recycling system. In order for blood to get back into the circulatory system after it goes through the spleen, most of it has to squeeze through tiny slits in the spleen's cords or sinuses. Old or damaged red blood cells don't compress easily, so they can't get through, and parasites and other detritus are pinched off the blood cells that do get through. This happens very smoothly and quickly, and the damaged junk is then recycled.

The spleen is surgically removed if it gets too big, if it's damaged by trauma, and in certain diseases such as Hodgkin's disease and some kinds of leukemia. Sickle cell anemia can destroy the spleen, and various diseases, congestive heart failure among them, can enlarge it to the point where leaving it in can be troublesome. Removal has consequences—it makes you more susceptible to infection, especially by bacteria, and especially if you are under twenty years old. In some cases, these infections can be overwhelming and fatal. But for most people, removing the spleen has little effect on the way the blood circulation system works, and you can go on living happily without it.

NOTES

1. By the Numbers

What Little Boys, Little Girls, and All the Rest of Us Are Made Of: Atomic composition chart from Robert A. Freitas, Jr., *Nanomedicine* (Austin, Texas: Landes Bioscience, 1999), www.foresight.org/Nanomedicine/Ch03_1.html.

Losing Our Hair: G. G. Schwartz and L. A. Rosenblu, "Allometry of Primate Hair Density and the Evolution of Human Hairlessness," *American Journal of Anthropology* 55 (1981): 9–12.

Vital Statistics: Gestational age data from U.S. Centers for Disease Control and Prevention, *Morbidity and Mortality Weekly Report* 56:14 (April 13, 2007): 344, www.cdc.gov/mmwr/preview/mmwrhtml/mm5614a7 .htm. Infant death data from U.S. Centers for Disease Control and Prevention, *Morbidity and Mortality Weekly Report* 56:42 (October 26, 2007): 1115, www.cdc.gov/mmwr/preview/mmwrhtml/mm5642a8 .htm. Based on preliminary data for 2005.

In Black and White: New York City birth weights in E. A. Howell et al., "Black/White Differences in Very Low Birth Weight Neonatal Mortality Rates Among New York City Hospitals," *Pediatrics* 121:3 (March 2008): 407–15. Opioid medicine discussed in M. Pletcher et al., "Trends in Opioid Prescribing by Race/Ethnicity for Patients Seeking Care in U.S. Emergency Departments," *Journal of the American Medical Association* 299:1 (January 2, 2008): 70–78. Cancer therapy disparities discussed in C. P. Gross et al., "Racial Disparities in Cancer Therapy," *Cancer* 112:4 (February 15, 2008): 900–908. Kidney transplants discussed in

D. Keith et al., "Insurance Type and Minority Status Associated with Large Disparities in Prelisting Dialysis Among Candidates for Kidney Transplantation," *Clinical Journal of the American Society of Nephrology* online, January 16, 2008, http://cjasn.asnjournals.org/cgi/rapidpdf/CJN.02220507v1.pdf. Mitral valve repairs covered in P. L. Digiorgi et al., "Mitral Valve Disease Presentation and Surgical Outcome in African-American Patients Compared with White Patients," *Annals of Thoracic Surgery* 85:1 (January 2008): 89–93. Soft tissue cancers described in S. Martinez et al., "Racial and Ethnic Differences in Treatment and Survival Among Adults with Primary Extremity Soft-tissue Sarcoma," *Cancer* 112:5 (March 1, 2008): 1162–68. Lung cancer surgery discussed in C. S. Lathan, B. A. Neville, and C. C. Earle, "The Effect of Race on Invasive Staging and Surgery in Non-small-cell Lung Cancer," *Journal of Clinical Oncology* 24:3 (January 20, 2006): 413–18. Lung transplants covered in D. J. Lederer et al., "Racial Differences in Waiting List Outcomes in Chronic Obstructive Pulmonary Disease," *American Journal of Respiratory and Critical Care Medicine* 177:4 (February 15, 2008): 450–54. Tobacco screening discussed in V. E. Cokkinides et al., "Racial and Ethnic Disparities in Smoking-cessation Interventions: Analysis of the 2005 National Health Interview Survey," *American Journal of Preventive Medicine* 34:5 (May 2008): 404–12. Breast cancer rates discussed in R. S. Levine et al., "Black-White Disparities in Elderly Breast Cancer Mortality Before and After Implementation of Medicare Benefits for Screening Mammography," *Journal of Health Care for the Poor and Underserved* 19:1 (2008). Breast cancer death rates covered in C. DeSantis et al., "Temporal Trends in Breast Cancer Mortality by State and Race," *Cancer Causes and Control* 19:5 (June 2008): 537–45. Rectal cancer discussed in A. M. Morris et al., "Residual Treatment Disparities After Oncology Referral for Rectal Cancer," *Journal of the National Cancer Institute* 100:10 (May 21, 2008): 738–44. Chronic kidney disease discussed in R. Mehrotra et al., "Racial Differences in Mortality Among Those with CKD," *Journal of the American Society of Nephrology* 19:7 (July 2008): 1403–10. Diabetes treatment disparities cited in T. D. Sequist, "Physician Performance and Racial Disparities in Diabetes Mellitus Care," *Archives of Internal Medicine* 168:11 (June 9, 2008): 1145–51. Death rate data from U.S. Centers for Disease Control and Prevention, *Morbidity and Mortality Weekly Report* 57:32 (August 15, 2008): 877, www.cdc.gov/mmwr/

preview/mmwrhtml/mm5732a6.htm. Based on preliminary data for 2006.

2. Butterflies in the Stomach

Real Diseases That Sound Like They Were Invented for a Horror Movie: All information on hemorrhagic fevers presented by the World Health Organization, www.who.int/en. Fungus infiltration discussed in Burkhard Bilger, "Letter from Oregon: The Mushroom Hunters," *New Yorker*, August 20, 2007, p. 62. Nicholas P. Money, *Mr. Bloomfield's Orchard: The Mysterious World of Mushrooms, Molds, and Mycologists* (New York: Oxford University Press, 2002).

Worms That Live Inside You: The information in this section comes largely from D. L. Kasper et al., eds., *Harrison's Principles of Internal Medicine*, 16th ed. (New York: McGraw-Hill, 2005). A. Salehabadi, G. Mowlavi, and S. M. Sadjjadi, "Human Infection with *Moniliformis moniliformis* in Iran: Another Case Report After Three Decades," *Vector-Borne and Zoonotic Diseases* 8:1 (2008): 101–3.

Maggot Therapy: Permissible amount of maggots in food products discussed in U.S. Food and Drug Administration, *Current Good Manufacturing Practices: Final Report*, August 9, 2004, section 1, p. 9, www.cfsan.fda.gov/~acrobat/gmp-1.pdf. Medicinal uses of maggots reported in Y. Nigam et al., "Maggot Therapy: The Science and Implication for CAM Part I—History and Bacterial Resistance," *Evidence-Based Complementary and Alternative Medicine* 3:2 (June 2006): 223–27.

Leech Me: Medicinal use of leeches reviewed in I. S. Whitaker et al., "By What Mechanism Do Leeches Help to Salvage Ischaemic Tissues? A Review," *British Journal of Oral and Maxillofacial Surgery* 43:2 (April 2005): 155–60. FDA approval of medicinal use of leeches reported in U.S. Food and Drug Administration, "FDA Clears Medicinal Leeches for Marketing," June 28, 2004, www.fda.gov/bbs/topics/answers/2004/ANS01294.html.

Evil Doctors and Nurses: Harold Shipman's story is summarized in Trevor Jackson and Richard Smith, "Harold Shipman, a General Practitioner and Murderer," *BMJ*, 328:7433 (January 24, 2004): 231. For Charles Cullen, see the collection of news articles at www.nj.com/news/cullen/. Michael Swango and evidence of wrongdoing discussed in James B. Stewart, *Blind Eye* (New York: Simon & Schuster, 1999). Murderer and medical student Karl Helge Hampus Svensson described in Lawrence Altman, "Swedes Ponder Whether Killer Can Be a Doctor," *New York Times*, January 25, 2008.

Can Your Hair Turn Gray Overnight?: Rhonda B. Graham, "The Science of Gray Hair," InteliHealth, last updated March 13, 2007, www.intelihealth.com/IH/ihtIH/WSIHW000/9023/24253/348513.html?d=dmtContent.

3. X, Y, and Sex

How Not to Improve Your Sex Life: List of "dietary supplements" sold as cures for erectile dysfunction reported in U.S. Food and Drug Administration, "Buying Fake ED Products Online," March 27, 2008, www.fda.gov/consumer/updates/erectiledysfunction010408.html. Recall requested for product with a potentially dangerous ingredient reported in U.S. Food and Drug Administration, "FDA Requests Recall of Xiadafil VIP Tabs," May 27, 2008, www.fda.gov/bbs/topics/NEWS/2008/NEW01840.html.

50 Percent: HPV infection rates from U.S. Centers for Disease Control and Prevention, *Morbidity and Mortality Weekly Report* 56:33 (August 24, 2007): 852, www.cdc.gov/mmwr/preview/mmwrhtml/mm5633a5.htm. National Health and Nutrition Examination Survey, 2003–2004.

Why Do Women Live Longer than Men?: Reasons for women living longer than men discussed in D. J. Kruger and R. M. Messe, "An Evolutionary Life-history Framework for Understanding Sex Differences in Human Mortality Rates," *Human Nature* 17:1 (Spring 2006): 74–97. Older research conducted on gendered mortality rates reviewed in T. H. Hollingworth, "A Demographic Study of the British Ducal Families," *Population Studies* 9 (1957): 4–26. Life expectancy data from U.S. Centers for Disease Control and Prevention, *Morbidity and Mortality Weekly Report* 56:51 (January 4, 2008): 1347, www.cdc.gov/mmwr/preview/mmwrhtml/mm5651a7.htm.

Why Women Get More Cavities than Men: John R. Lukacs, "Fertility and Agriculture Accentuate Sex Differences in Dental Caries Rates," *Current Anthropology* 49:5 (2008): 901–14.

Rotten Luck: U.S. Centers for Disease Control and Prevention, *Morbidity and Mortality Weekly Report* 56:32 (August 17, 2007): 823, www.cdc.gov/mmwr/preview/mmwrhtml/mm5632a6.htm.

Will It Be a Boy or a Girl?: Family-tree research presented in C. Gellarly, "Trends in Population Sex Ratios May Be Explained by Changes in the Frequencies of Polymorphic Alleles of a Sex Ratio Gene," *Evolutionary Biology* online, December 13, 2008, www.springerlink.com/content/d87k212rx717211g/, by subscription.

Don't Blame Breast-feeding: Cause of drooping breasts discussed in B. Rinker, M. Veneracion, and C. P. Walsh, "The Effect of Breastfeeding on Breast Aesthetics," *Aesthetic Surgery* 28:5 (September 2008): 534–37. Percentage breast-fed data from U.S. Centers for Disease Control and Prevention, *Morbidity and Mortality Weekly Report* 55:42 (October 27, 2006): 1155, www.cdc.gov/mmwr/preview/mmwrhtml/mm5542a6.htm. Data 2002 National Survey of Family Growth.

4. Bedside Manner

What's Inside an Ambulance?: "Part-800 Equipment Inventory," Policy Statement No. 98-14, issued by John J. Clair, Bureau of Emergency Medical Services, New York State Department of Health, October 15, 1998, www.health.state.ny.us/nysdoh/ems/pdf/9814.pdf.

Why Is It Called a Charley (or Charlie) Horse?: Mencken as possible source discussed in H. B. Woolf, "Mencken as Etymologist: Charley Horse and Lobster Trick," *American Speech* 48:3/4 (Autumn–Winter, 1973): 229–38. Earlier use of the term discussed in D. Shulman, "Whence 'Charley Horse'?" *American Speech* 24:2 (April 1949): 100–104.

5. Lab Rat

Of Mice and Men: D. Nguyen and T. Xu, "The Expanding Role of Mouse Genetics for Understanding Human Biology and Disease," *Disease Models & Mechanisms* 1 (July 2008): 56–66.

The Trouble with Twins: D. Boomsma, A. Busjahn, and L. Peltonen, "Classical Twin Studies and Beyond," *Nature Reviews Genetics* 3:11 (2002): 872–82.

Can I Donate Blood?: The study referred to is B. Newman and S. Graves, "A Study of 178 Consecutive Vasovagal Syncopal Reactions from the Perspective of Safety," *Transfusion* 41:12 (2001): 1475–79.

6. Biohazard!

The World's Six Worst Infectious Diseases: Statistics from the World Health Organization, www.who.int/en/, and U.S. Centers for Disease Control and Prevention, www.cdc.gov/.

Ten Diseases You Can Get from Your Dog or Your Cat: P. M. Rabinowitz et al., "Pet-Related Infections," *American Family Physician* 76 (2007): 1314–22.

Exotic and Deadly: Dangers of exotic pets reported in L. K. Pickering et al., Committee on Infectious Diseases, "Exposure to Nontraditional Pets at Home and to Animals in Public Settings: Risks to Children," *Pediatrics* 122:4 (October 2008): 876–86. List of human pathogens reported in L. H. Taylor et al., "Risk Factors for Human Disease Emergence," *Philosophical Transactions of the Royal Society of London B: Biological Sciences* 356:1411 (2001): 983–89. Diseases caught from zoo reptiles discussed in C. R. Friedman et al., "An Outbreak of Salmonellosis Among Children Attending a Reptile Exhibit at a Zoo," *Journal of Pediatrics* 132:5 (1998): 802–7.

The Twenty-four Vaccine-Preventable Diseases: "Vaccines & Preventable Diseases," U.S. Centers for Disease Control and Prevention, Department of Health and Human Services, updated July 19, 2007, www.cdc .gov/vaccines/vpd-vac/default.htm.

7. The Perfect Cure

Take Two and Call in the Morning: Edmund Stone, "An Account of the Success of the Bark of the Willow in the Cure of Agues," *Philosophical Transactions* 53 (1763), 195–200.

Reduce Your Risk by Drinking Coffee . . . : The relationship between Type 2 diabetes and coffee studied in Rob M. van Dam and Frank B. Hu, "Coffee Consumption and Risk of Type 2 Diabetes: A Systematic Review," *Journal of the American Medical Association* 294:1 (July 6, 2005): 97–104. See also B. Smith et al., "Does Coffee Consumption Reduce the Risk of Type 2 Diabetes in Individuals with Impaired Glucose?" *Diabetes Care* 29:11 (November 2006): 2385–90. High blood pressure and coffee discussed in Cuno S.P.M. Uiterwaal et al., "Coffee Intake and Incidence of Hypertension," *American Journal of Clinical Nutrition* 85:3 (March 2007): 718–23. Alcoholic cirrhosis and coffee reviewed in S. F. Kendrick and C. P. Day, "A Coffee with Your Brandy, Sir?" *Journal of Hepatology* 46:5 (May 2007): 980–82. Liver cancer and coffee studied in Keitaro Tanaka et al., "Inverse Association Between Coffee Drinking and the Risk of Hepatocellular Carcinoma: A Case-control Study in Japan," *Cancer Science* 98:2 (February 2007): 214–18. Heart disease and coffee researched in M. C. Cornelis and A. El-Sohemy,

"Coffee, Caffeine, and Coronary Heart Disease," *Current Opinion in Lipidology* 18:1 (February 2007): 13–19.

. . . *or Drinking Alcohol:* Renal cancer and alcohol discussed in Jung Eun Lee et al., "Alcohol Intake and Renal Cell Cancer in a Pooled Analysis of 12 Prospective Studies," *Journal of the National Cancer Institute* 99 (2007): 801–10. Heart attacks and alcohol discussed in W. J. Joline, "Alcohol Consumption and Risk for Coronary Heart Disease Among Men with Hypertension," *Annals of Internal Medicine* 146:1 (2007): 10–19. See also J. Kenneth et al., "Alcohol Consumption and Risk for Coronary Heart Disease in Men with Healthy Lifestyles," *Archives of Internal Medicine* 166 (2006): 2145–50. Women, heart attacks, and alcohol studied in Joan M. Dorn et al., "Alcohol Drinking Pattern and Non-fatal Myocardial Infarction in Women," *Addiction* 102 (2007): 730–39. Heart failure and alcohol researched in Chris L. Bryson et al., "The Association of Alcohol Consumption and Incident Heart Failure: The Cardiovascular Health Study," *Journal of the American College of Cardiology* 48 (2006): 305–11.

The Cranberry Juice Cure: R. G. Jepson and J. C. Craig, "Cranberries for Preventing Urinary Tract Infections," *Cochrane Database of Systematic Reviews* 23:1 (2008), article number CD001321.

Why Chocolate Is Good for You: Chocolate, antioxidants, and cardiovascular disease reviewed in G. Lippi et al., "Dark Chocolate: Consumption for Pleasure or Therapy?" *Journal of Thrombosis and Thrombolysis* 23 (September 2008): 1–7. Chocolate and blood pressure discussed in D. Taubert, R. Roesen, and E. Schömig, "Effect of Cocoa and Tea Intake on Blood Pressure: A Meta-analysis," *Archives of Internal Medicine* 167:7 (April 9, 2007): 626–34.

Why Garlic Is Good for You: G. A. Benavides et al., "Hydrogen Sulfide Mediates the Vasoactivity of Garlic," *Proceedings of the National Academy of Sciences of the United States of America* 104:46 (November 13, 2007): 17977–82.

8. Prevention Is the Best Medicine

Poisoned: U.S. Centers for Disease Control and Prevention, "QuickStats: Death Rates from Poisoning, by State—United States, 2004," *Morbidity and Mortality Weekly Report* 56:36 (September 14, 2007): 938, www.cdc.gov/mmwr/preview/mmwrhtml/mm5636a6.htm. See also U.S. Centers for Disease Control and Prevention, "Compressed Mortality

File: Underlying Cause-of-Death," Wide-ranging Online Data for Epidemiologic Research, http://wonder.cdc.gov/mortsql.html.

Thank You for Not Smoking: For the full 910-page report, see U.S. Office of the Surgeon General, "The Health Consequences of Smoking: 2004 Surgeon General's Report," www.cdc.gov/tobacco/data_statistics/sgr/sgr_2004/chapters.htm. See also the report on secondhand smoke, U.S. Office of the Surgeon General, "The Health Consequences of Involuntary Exposure to Tobacco Smoke: A Report of the Surgeon General," 2006, www.surgeongeneral.gov/library/secondhandsmoke/report. Sleep problems and smoking, American College of Physicians, "Smoking Linked to Sleep Disturbances: Nightly Nicotine Withdrawal May Contribute to Restless Sleep," *Chest,* press release, February 2008.

Secondhand Smoke: M. Maria Glymour et al., "Spousal Smoking and Incidence of First Stroke: The Health and Retirement Study," *American Journal of Preventive Medicine* 35:3 (September 2008): 245–48.

Can You Prevent Your Skin from Wrinkling? G. J. Fisher, J. Varani, and J. J. Voorhees, "Looking Older: Fibroblast Collapse and Therapeutic Implications," *Archives of Dermatology* 144:5 (May 2008): 666–72.

Who Gets Bitten by Venomous Snakes? The number of snakebites per year is estimated in A. Kasturiratne et al., "The Global Burden of Snakebite: A Literature Analysis and Modelling Based on Regional Estimates of Envenoming and Deaths," *PLoS Medicine* online, 4:5 (November 2008): e218. Snakebite cases within the United States reviewed in Willis A. Wingert and Linda Chan, "Rattlesnake Bites in Southern California and Rationale for Recommended Treatment West," *Western Journal of Medicine* 148:1 (January 1988): 37–44.

Unhealthful Behavior: U.S. Centers for Disease Control and Prevention, *Morbidity and Mortality Weekly Report* 56:4 (February 2, 2007): 79, www.cdc.gov/mmwr/preview/mmwrhtml/mm5604a5.htm.

Who Doesn't Get Enough Exercise? U.S. Centers for Disease Control and Prevention, "Prevalence of Regular Physical Activity Among Adults—United States, 2001 and 2005," *Morbidity and Mortality Weekly Report* 56:46 (November 23, 2007): 1209–12, www.cdc.gov/mmwr/preview/mmwrhtml/mm5646a1.htm.

Watching Their Weight: U.S. Centers for Disease Control and Prevention, *Morbidity and Mortality Weekly Report* 55:45 (November 17, 2006): 1229, www.cdc.gov/mmwr/preview/mmwrhtml/mm5545a5.htm.

Jobs That Are Bad for Your Health: U.S. Bureau of Labor Statistics, "Table 2. Fatal Occupational Injuries by Industry and Selected Event or Exposure, 2007," Census of Fatal Occupational Injuries Summary 2007, August 20, 2008, www.bls.gov/news.release/cfoi.t02.htm.

9. Invention Is the Best Medicine

Medical Firsts: Cesarean birthrate data from U.S. Centers for Disease Control and Prevention, *Morbidity and Mortality Weekly Report* 56:15 (April 20, 2007): 373, www.cdc.gov/mmwr/preview/mmwrhtml/mm5615a8 .htm. Based on preliminary data for 2005. Artificial insemination discussed in R. H. Foote, "The History of Artificial Insemination: Selected Notes and Notables," *Journal of Animal Science,* electronic supplement 2, 2002, www.asas.org/symposia/esupp2/Footehist.pdf.

Thirty People Who Probably Like Having a Disease Named After Them . . . : The frequently updated Web site www.whonamedit.com/ is a good source for medical eponyms but, good as it is, it's not complete.

Hometown Germs: D. T. Dennis et al., "Tularemia as a Biological Weapon: Medical and Public Health Management," *Journal of the American Medical Association* 285:21 (June 6, 2001): 2763–73.

10. Scared to Death

Can You Be Scared to Death? Death from strong emotions reviewed in G. L. Engel, "Sudden and Rapid Death During Psychological Stress," *Annals of Internal Medicine* 74 (1971): 771–82. Animal cases of heart attack and death discussed in Martin A. Samuels, "The Brain-Heart Connection," *Circulation* 116:1 (July 3, 2007): 77–84. Anxiety as a factor in mortality reviewed in G. A. Brenes et al., "Scared to Death: Results from the Health, Aging, and Body Composition Study," *American Journal of Geriatric Psychiatry* 15:3 (March 2007): 262–65.

Can You Be Scared Stiff? A. K. Moskowitz, " 'Scared Stiff': Catatonia as an Evolutionary-based Fear Response," *Psychological Review* 111:4 (October 2004): 984–1002.

Catching Our Breath: U.S. Centers for Disease Control and Prevention, *Morbidity and Mortality Weekly Report* 56:45 (November 16, 2007): 1193, www.cdc.gov/mmwr/preview/mmwrhtml/mm5645a6.htm.

Can You Die of a Broken Heart? I. S. Wittstein, "Acute Stress Cardiomyopathy," *Current Heart Failure Reports* 5:2 (June 2008): 61–68.

Good for the Heart: U.S. Centers for Disease Control and Prevention,

Morbidity and Mortality Weekly Report 56:26 (July 6, 1007): 659, www.cdc.gov/mmwr/preview/mmwrhtml/mm5626a5.htm.

The Top Ten Killers: Diseases and U.S. fatalities reported in U.S. Centers for Disease Control and Prevention, *National Vital Statistics Reports* 56:10 (April 24, 2008). The 2005 figures are the latest available as of this writing. Diabetes as cause of death reviewed in Hsiang-Ching Kung et al., U.S. Centers for Disease Control and Prevention, "Table B. Percentage of Total Deaths, Death Rates, and Age-adjusted Death Rates for 2005, Percentage Change in Age-adjusted Death Rates from 2004 to 2005, and Ratio of Age-adjusted Death Rates by Race and Sex in 2005, for the 15 Leading Causes of Death for the Total Population: United States," *National Vital Statistics Reports* 56:10 (April 2008): 5.

What Are You Most Likely to Die Of?: Hsiang-Ching Kung, U.S. Centers for Disease Control and Prevention, "Deaths: Final Data for 2005," *National Vital Statistics Report* 56:10 (April 2008): 1–121.

Death by Accident: U.S. Centers for Disease Control and Prevention, *Morbidity and Mortality Weekly Report* 57:25 (June 27, 2008): 701, www.cdc.gov/mmwr/preview/mmwrhtml/mm5725a7.htm.

Which Is More Common, Suicide or Homicide? U.S. Centers for Disease Control and Prevention, *Morbidity and Mortality Weekly Report* 56:25 (June 29, 2007): 635, www.cdc.gov/mmwr/preview/mmwrhtml/mm5625a5.htm.

Death by Natural Disaster: K. A. Borden and S. L. Cutter, "Spatial Patterns of Natural Hazards Mortality in the United States," *International Journal of Health Geographics* 7:1 (December 17, 2008): 64.

11. Gray Matter

Why Do We Need Sleep?: U.S. Centers for Disease Control and Prevention, *Morbidity and Mortality Weekly Report* 57:8 (February 29, 2008): 209, www.cdc.gov/mmwr/preview/mmwrhtml/mm5708a8.htm.

Left- and Right-Handedness: Handedness categories reviewed in M. K. Holder, *Hand Preference Questionnaires: One Gets What One Asks For,* M. Phil. thesis, Department of Anthropology, Rutgers University, New Brunswick, N.J., 1992. Gender as factor in twins studied in Syuichi Ooki, "Genetic and Environmental Influences on the Handedness and Footedness in Japanese Twin Children," *Twin Research and Human Genetics* 8:6 (December 2005): 649–56(8). Asymmetry in the brain studied in J. C. McManus, *Right Hand, Left Hand: The Origins of*

Asymmetry in Brains, Bodies, Atoms and Cultures (London: Weidenfeld and Nicolson, 2002).

So How Come They Can't Do Long Division?: B. Bloom and R. A. Cohen, "Summary Health Statistics for U.S. Children: National Health Interview Survey, 2006," *Vital Health Statistics* 10:234 (2007), www.cdc .gov/nchs/nhis.htm.

Why Teenagers Act Nuts: Logical skills versus psychosocial maturity discussed in Laurence Steinberg, "Risk Taking in Adolescence," *Current Directions in Psychological Science* 16:2 (2007): 55–59. The fMRI research is reported in A. Baird et al., " 'What Were You Thinking?' An fMRI Study of Adolescent Decision Making," poster presented at the annual meeting of the Cognitive Neuroscience Society, April 2005.

12. An Appendix

Is the Appendix Really Useless?: R. Randal Bollinger et al., "Biofilms in the Large Bowel Suggest an Apparent Function of the Human Vermiform Appendix," *Journal of Theoretical Biology* 249:4 (December 21, 2007): 826–31. M. J. Burton and P. P. Glasziou, "Tonsillectomy or Adeno-tonsillectomy versus Non-surgical Treatment for Chronic/Recurrent Acute Tonsillitis," *Cochrane Database of Systematic Reviews*, January 21, 2009.

ACKNOWLEDGMENTS

My thanks for many helpful suggestions to the following: James Bakalar; Kenneth Bakalar; Stanley Bone, MD; Maureen Empfield, MD; Scott Kirsch, MD; Bonnie Kirsch; Linda Lewis, MD; Eric Marcus, MD; Neesha Patel, MD; Steven Roose, MD; and Milton Wainberg, MD.

Yet again, a book of mine would not exist without the generous attention of John Thornton, my agent and friend, who had the original idea for this book and guided the project from start to finish.

Robin Dennis, my editor, and her assistant, Emi Ikkanda, may well be two of the hardest-working people in book publishing. And I am lucky to have had the sharp-eyed Emily DeHuff as my copy editor.

The patient attention and helpful advice of my wife, Francine Cournos, MD, was essential in this book, as it is for me in everything.

ILLUSTRATION CREDITS

Stapes and penny: Courtesy of Otolaryngology Houston, www.ghorayeb.com.

Biohazard research suit for work with Ebola and other viruses: Photo by James Gathany, 2007. Courtesy of the CDC, Public Health Image Library image 10723.

Maggots in a wound: Courtesy of Volker Steger/Photo Researchers, Inc.

Green bottle fly: Courtesy of Colin L. Miller, Tucson, Arizona, www.colinlmiller.com.

Harold Shipman: Photo by Greater Manchester Police. Courtesy of *The New York Times* Archives.

World War II ambulance training: Courtesy of Otis Historical Archives, National Museum of Health and Medicine.

Jim Lonborg: Photo by Barton Silverman. Courtesy of *The New York Times* Archives.

Sir Arthur Conan Doyle: George Grantham Bain Collection, Library of Congress, LC-B2-2614-9.

Knockout mouse: Courtesy of the National Human Genome Research Institute.

Sir Francis Galton: Photo by the studio of Elliott & Fry, London. Courtesy of *The New York Times* Archives.

Malaria public notice: Courtesy of Otis Historical Archives, National Museum of Health and Medicine.

Prairie dog: Photo by Kevin Molonkey / *The New York Times*.

Statue of smallpox god: Photo by James Gathany, 2005. Courtesy of the

U.S. Centers for Disease Control and Prevention, Public Health Image Library image 8003.

Hiccups cure: U.S. Patent Office, patent no. 7062320, June 13, 2006.

Carolina pygmy rattlesnake: Photo by John Willson, Savannah River Ecology Laboratory, 2005. Courtesy of the U.S. Centers for Disease Control and Prevention, Public Health Image Library image 8138.

Lobstering: Photo by Nicole Bengiveno / *The New York Times*.

Caesar: From *The Museum of Antiquity* by L. W. Yaggy and T. L. Haines, 1882.

First artificial leg: Courtesy of the Science Museum, London.

Testicular implant mechanism: U.S. Patent Office, patent no. 5653757, August 15, 1997.

Dr. Cushing's cake: Courtesy of Yale University, Harvey Cushing / John Hay Whitney Medical Library.

Guillaume Duchenne: From his book *Mécanisme de la physionomie humaine* (1862).

Old Lyme, Connecticut: Photo by Emily S. Rueb / *The New York Times*.

Passengers disembarking from cruise ship after discovery of Norwalk virus: Photo by Ting-Li Wang / *The New York Times*.

Castor plant: Photo by Rob Cardillo / *The New York Times*.

INDEX

Page numbers in *italics* refer to illustrations.

About the Author

NICHOLAS BAKALAR contributes the "Vital Signs" column to *The New York Times*. The author or co-author of twelve books, including *Where the Germs Are: A Scientific Safari,* he also writes for *Discover* magazine and *Wildlife Conservation.* He lives in New York City.

Printed in the USA
CPSIA information can be obtained
at www.ICGtesting.com
LVHW091132150724
785511LV00001B/90

9 780805 088540